HANI
CC
ORTH
FRACTURES

Fourth Edition

Scott Hal Kozin, M.D.
Assistant Professor of Orthopaedic Surgery
Temple University School of Medicine
Philadelphia, Pennsylvania

Anthony Clayton Berlet, M.D.
Assistant Clinical Professor
Department of Plastic and Reconstructive Surgery
UMDNJ - New Jersey Medical School
Newark, New Jersey

2000

HANDBOOK OF COMMON ORTHOPAEDIC FRACTURES

Fourth Edition

Illustrations by Anthony C. Berlet, M.D.

PREFACE

Orthopaedic surgery is a field of medicine that encompasses a wide spectrum of disease entities and fractures. Fractures may occur anywhere in the human and accurate assessment is essential for diagnosis and treatment. Fractures throughout the body have been extensively analyzed and classified. These classifications are based on fracture configurations, mechanism of injury or fracture stability. This has led to an overwhelming number of classifications and eponyms which are frequently confusing and cumbersome. In addition, many fractures have multiple classifications creating further confusion. A classification should provide therapeutic and prognostic information to be valuable in fracture management.

The Fourth Edition of the **HANDBOOK OF COMMON ORTHOPAEDIC FRACTURES** is published for the practicing physician, resident, medical student and other health care professionals to simplify fracture classifications, help access fracture stability, and direct treatment. All fractures should initially be described according to length, angulation, rotation, displacement, and degree of comminution, prior to attempting specific classification. These variables are essential in orthopaedic analysis for treatment of fractures and are incorporated in many of the classification schemas. This handbook contains the majority of fractures that have been appropriately classified and includes an Eponym section for reference purposes. Extremely uncommon fractures and those without adequate classification are not included in this text.

This handbook is organized into seven sections: (1) Upper Extremity, (2) Spine, (3) Pelvis and Acetabulum, (4) Lower Extremity, (5) Pediatrics, and (6) Osteonecrosis and Osteochondrosis and (7) Eponyms. The fracture classifications are listed in a distal to proximal direction for the Upper Extremity followed by a cephalad to caudad direction for the remaining sections. The Eponym section is listed in alphabetical order and includes adult and pediatric nomenclature. This organization is designed to allow quick and easy reference to specific fracture classifications.

The **HANDBOOK OF COMMON ORTHOPAEDIC FRACTURES, Fourth Edition**, is physically designed to fit in a pocket to allow for easy accessibility. We hope this text will be useful in simplifying fracture assessment and classifications. We continue to welcome any suggestions, comments, and criticisms that may improve our handbook.

We wish to thank Edward J. Barbieri, Ph.D., and G. John DiGregorio, M.D., Ph.D., for their assistance with the composition and preparation of this handbook.

Scott H. Kozin, M.D.
Anthony C. Berlet, M.D.

TABLE OF CONTENTS

INTRODUCTION

Orthopaedic fracture management begins with initial patient evaluation. The entire patient and involved extremity should be carefully and thoroughly examined. A complete neurovascular examination of the potentially fractured extremity is vital in the initial assessment. Neurovascular compromise is an orthopaedic emergency and requires prompt therapeutic intervention. All fractures should be initially splinted to prevent further tissue damage and for patient comfort. The skin should be inspected for evidence of bone penetration leading to open fracture management. Open fractures require cultures, debridement, antibiotics, and sterile dressings as part of their initial management. Radiographic analysis should be prompt and should include the joint above and below the fracture; for example, a femoral shaft fracture should have radiographic visualization of the entire femur including the femoral head and condyles.

After careful history, physical examination, and radiography, an appropriate description of the fracture should be formulated. Orthopaedic fracture description is based upon length, angulation, rotation, and degree of bony comminution. A fractured extremity may be shortened or distracted, angulated in multiple directions, malrotated, or severely comminuted. All of these factors influence the therapeutic decision process and effect overall prognosis. Fractures should also be described as open with bone penetration of the skin or closed with preservation of the overlying skin. Fracture description should include the overlying soft tissue damage as well as the disruption of underlying bone and neurovascular elements. These variables all are indicative of the amount of energy absorbed by the fractured extremity at the time of injury. These factors are major determinants in the overall prognosis of the injured extremity.

Many fractures have been organized into classification schemas to provide therapeutic and prognostic information valuable in fracture management. This third edition text organizes those orthopaedic classifications into six expanded sections:

      (1)   Upper Extremity,
      (2)   Spine,
      (3)   Pelvis and Acetabulum,
      (4)   Lower Extremity, and
      (5)   Pediatrics.
      (6)   Osteonecrosis and Osteochondrosis

The Upper Extremity classifications are listed in a distal to proximal direction beginning with distal phalangeal fractures and progressing proximally including Frykman's classification of wrist fractures, Mason's classifications of radial head fractures, and Neer's classification of proximal humeral fractures. Each fracture classification is accompanied by extensive illustrations to aid in the understanding and application of specific classification schemas.

The Spine section progresses from a cephalad to caudad direction and includes cervical and thoracolumbar fractures. There is a separate section dedicated to odontoid fractures with illustrations in both the anteroposterior and lateral views.

The third section concentrates on pelvis and acetabular fractures. Tile's classification of pelvic disruption and acetabular fractures was selected because of its valuable therapeutic and prognostic information. This classification is presented in outline form with detailed illustrations to simplify its application in the clinical setting.

The fourth section involves the entire lower extremity beginning with hip fractures. These fractures are divided into femoral neck, intertrochanteric and subtrochanteric classifications. Accurate classification of these common fractures is necessary to select appropriate treatment. This section lists fractures in a superior to inferior direction and includes Winquist's classification of femoral shaft comminution, Hawkin's classification of talar neck fractures, and Essex-Lopresti's classification of calcaneus fractures. Ankle fractures are commonly classified according to either the Lauge-Hansen or Danis-Weber schema. Therefore, both of these classifications are included in this text.

The fifth section discusses pediatric fractures beginning with the Salter-Harris classification of physeal disruptions. This classification is used to describe the majority of pediatric fractures. Additional specific upper and lower extremity schemas are presented to complete this section.

The new sixth section concerns the topics osteonecrosis and osteochondrosis. The diagnosis of osteonecrosis indicates that the ischemic death of bone and marrow has occurred. The diagnosis of osteochondrosis initially was interpreted as primary impairment of local blood supply that led to a similar sequence as osteonecrosis. However, further investigation into osteochondrosis has determined that many cases of ostechondrosis do not have histologic evidence of dead bone. Therefore, these two entities overlap and are included in a single section that describes this heterogeneous group of disorders.

The seventh section of this handbook is dedicated to fracture eponyms. Eponyms to describe various fracture configurations are commonly employed. An alphabetical listing of fracture eponyms with illustrations and references is presented to allow easy accessibility.

The organization into these various sections is to allow an easily accessible reference text to specific fracture classifications and eponyms. The detailed illustrations are to simplify the understanding of these classification schemas. Hopefully, this combination of text and illustrations will simplify orthopaedic fracture classifications and be useful in the clinical setting.

UPPER EXTREMITY

DISTAL PHALANX FRACTURES

(Kaplan Classification)

I.   LONGITUDINAL

II.   TRANSVERSE

III. COMMINUTED

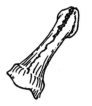

I. Longitudinal

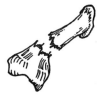

II. Transverse

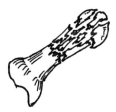

III. Comminuted

BASE OF THUMB METACARPAL FRACTURES

(Green Classification)

INTRA-ARTICULAR FRACTURES

      I.   BENNETT'S FRACTURE

      II.   ROLANDO'S FRACTURE

EXTRA-ARTICULAR FRACTURES

      III.   FRACTURES OF THE METACARPAL BASE

           A.   TRANSVERSE

           B.   OBLIQUE

      IV.   EPIPHYSEAL FRACTURE

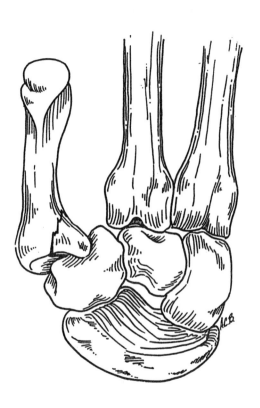

BASE OF THUMB METACARPAL FRACTURES

(Green Classification)

INTRA-ARTICULAR FRACTURES

      I.   BENNETT'S FRACTURE

      II.   ROLANDO'S FRACTURE

BENNETT'S and ROLANDO's FRACTURES are further described in the EPONYM SECTION.

I. Bennett's
   Fracture

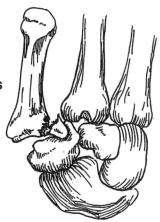

II. Rolando's
    Fracture

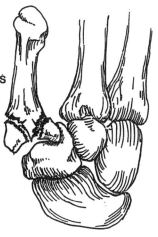

9

BASE OF THUMB METACARPAL FRACTURES

(Green Classification)

EXTRA-ARTICULAR FRACTURES

    III.   FRACTURES OF THE METACARPAL BASE

          A.   TRANSVERSE

          B.   OBLIQUE

    IV.   EPIPHYSEAL FRACTURE

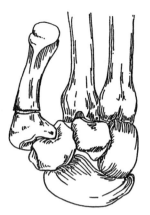

IIIA. Transverse

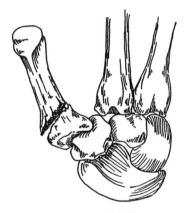

IIIB. Oblique

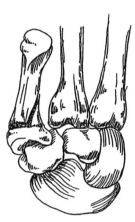

IV. Epiphyseal

SCAPHOID FRACTURES

(Russe Classification)

ANATOMIC LOCATION

    I.   PROXIMAL THIRD - 20%[a]

    II.   MIDDLE THIRD - 70%

    III.   DISTAL THIRD - 10%

FRACTURE CONFIGURATION

    I.   TRANSVERSE

    II.   VERTICAL OBLIQUE

    III.   HORIZONTAL OBLIQUE

Proximal third scaphoid fractures have increased incidence of avascular necrosis.

Forces across the wrist tend to compress and stabilize the horizontal oblique and transverse scaphoid fractures. The vertical oblique configuration tends to displace as the forces shear the fracture surface.

[a] *Percentages indicate the frequency of fracture occurrence.*

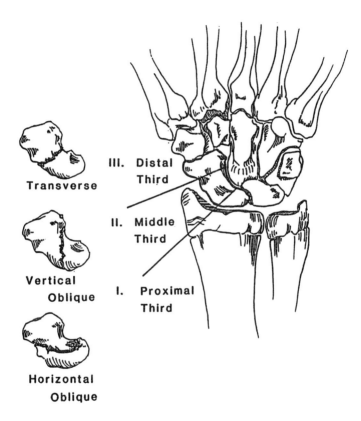

Transverse

Vertical Oblique

Horizontal Oblique

III. Distal Third

II. Middle Third

I. Proximal Third

FRACTURES OF THE DISTAL RADIUS

(Frykman Classification)

FRACTURE PATTERN	DISTAL ULNA FRACTURE	
	ABSENT	PRESENT
EXTRA-ARTICULAR	I	II
INTRA-ARTICULAR INVOLVING RADIOCARPAL JOINT	III	IV
INTRA-ARTICULAR INVOLVING RADIOULNAR JOINT	V	VI
INTRA-ARTICULAR INVOLVING RADIOCARPAL and RADIOULNAR JOINTS	VII	VIII

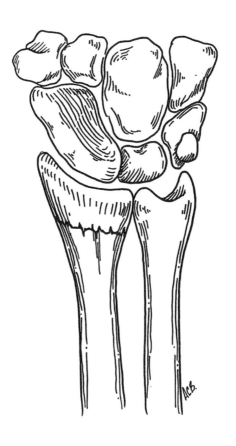

FRACTURES OF THE DISTAL RADIUS

(Frykman Classification)

FRACTURE PATTERN	DISTAL ULNA FRACTURE	
	ABSENT	PRESENT
EXTRA-ARTICULAR	I	II
INTRA-ARTICULAR INVOLVING RADIOCARPAL JOINT	III	IV

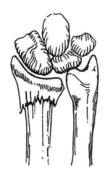

I.

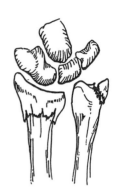

II.

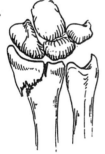

III.

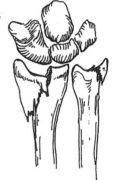

IV.

FRACTURES OF THE DISTAL RADIUS

(Frykman Classification)

FRACTURE PATTERN	DISTAL ULNA FRACTURE	
	ABSENT	PRESENT
INTRA-ARTICULAR INVOLVING RADIOULNAR JOINT	V	VI
INTRA-ARTICULAR INVOLVING RADIOCARPAL and RADIOULNAR JOINTS	VII	VIII

V.

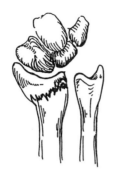

VI.

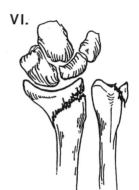

VII.

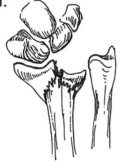

VIII.

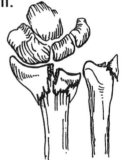

FRACTURES OF THE PROXIMAL ULNA
WITH RADIAL HEAD DISLOCATION - MONTEGGIA LESION

(Bado Classification)

I.   ANTERIOR DISLOCATION OF THE RADIAL HEAD AND FRACTURE OF
     THE ULNAR DIAPHYSIS AT ANY LEVEL WITH ANTERIOR
     ANGULATION

II. POSTERIOR OR POSTEROLATERAL DISLOCATION OF THE RADIAL
     HEAD AND FRACTURE OF THE ULNAR DIAPHYSIS WITH
     POSTERIOR ANGULATION

III. LATERAL OR ANTEROLATERAL DISLOCATION OF THE RADIAL HEAD
     AND FRACTURE OF THE ULNAR METAPHYSIS

IV. ANTERIOR DISLOCATION OF THE RADIAL HEAD, FRACTURE OF THE
     THE PROXIMAL THIRD OF THE RADIUS, AND FRACTURE OF THE
     THE ULNA AT THE SAME LEVEL

*Type I fracture dislocation is the most common type, accounting for
approximately 65 percent of Monteggia lesions. Type IV lesions are uncommon, less
than 5 percent of total.*

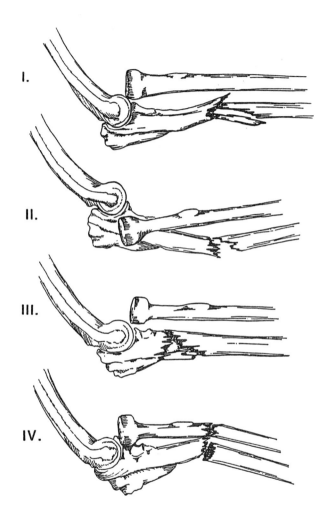

I.

II.

III.

IV.

CLASSIFICATION OF OLECRANON FRACTURES

(Morrey Classification)

I. UNDISPLACED

    A. NONCOMMINUTED

    B. COMMINUTED

II. DISPLACED - STABLE

    A. NONCOMMINUTED

    B. COMMINUTED

III. DISPLACED - UNSTABLE

    A. NONCOMMINUTED

    B. COMMINUTED

The higher fracture types have less satisfactory results.

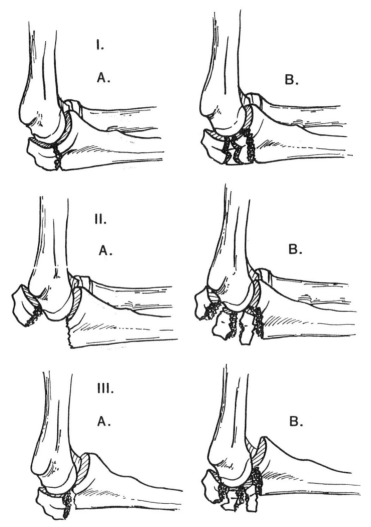

CORONOID FRACTURES

(Morrey Classification)

I.   AVULSION OF THE TIP OF THE CORONOID PROCESS

II.   SINGLE OR COMMINUTED FRAGMENT INVOLVING 50 PERCENT OR LESS OF THE CORONOID PROCESS

III.   SINGLE OR COMMINUTED FRAGMENT INVOLVING GREATER THAN 50 PERCENT OF THE CORONOID PROCESS

Coronoid fractures are uncommon and often associated with elbow dislocations.

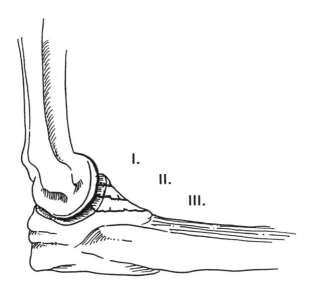

I.

II.

III.

FRACTURES OF THE RADIAL HEAD

(Mason Classification with Johnston Modification)

I. NONDISPLACED LINEAR OR TRANSVERSE FRACTURES - 50%[a]

II. FRACTURES WITH MINIMAL DISPLACEMENT OR COMMINUTED
FRACTURES WITHOUT DISPLACEMENT - 20%

III. COMMINUTED FRACTURES WITH MARKED DISPLACEMENT - 20%

IV. RADIAL HEAD FRACTURES WITH ELBOW DISLOCATION - 10%

Most common elbow fracture in adults.

[a] *Percentages indicate the frequency of fracture occurrence.*

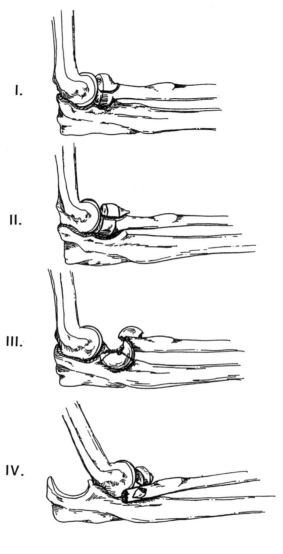

I.

II.

III.

IV.

FRACTURES OF THE DISTAL HUMERUS

(Muller Classification)

A. **EXTRA-ARTICULAR FRACTURES**

    A1. AVULSION FRACTURES OF THE EPICONDYLES

    A2. SIMPLE SUPRACONDYLAR FRACTURE

    A3. COMMINUTED SUPRACONDYLAR FRACTURE

B. **INTRA-ARTICULAR FRACTURES OF ONE CONDYLE**

    B1. FRACTURE OF THE TROCHLEA

    B2. FRACTURE OF THE CAPITELLUM

    B3. TANGENTIAL FRACTURE OF THE TROCHLEA

C. **BI-CONDYLAR FRACTURES**

    C1. Y-FRACTURE

    C2. Y-FRACTURE WITH SUPRACONDYLAR COMMINUTION

    C3. COMMINUTED FRACTURE

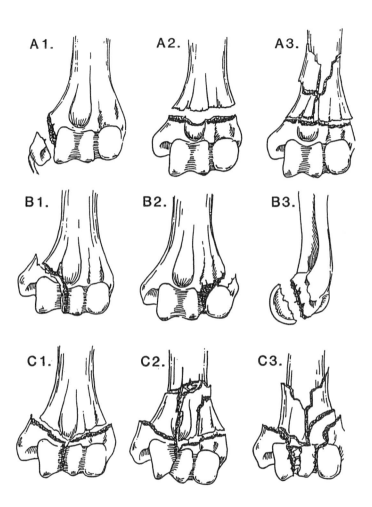

FRACTURES OF THE HUMERAL CONDYLES

(Milch Classification)

LATERAL HUMERAL CONDYLE

I.   SIMPLE FRACTURE OF THE LATERAL CONDYLE WITH LATERAL WALL
      OF TROCHLEA ATTACHED TO MAIN MASS OF THE HUMERUS

II.   FRACTURE WITH LATERAL WALL OF TROCHLEA ATTACHED TO
      FRACTURED LATERAL CONDYLAR FRAGMENT

MEDIAL LATERAL CONDYLE

I.   SIMPLE FRACTURE OF MEDIAL CONDYLE WITH LATERAL WALL OF
      TROCHLEA ATTACHED TO MAIN MASS OF THE HUMERUS

II.   FRACTURE WITH LATERAL WALL OF TROCHLEA ATTACHED TO
      FRACTURED MEDIAL CONDYLAR FRAGMENT

Type II fractures involve the trochlea and are unstable.

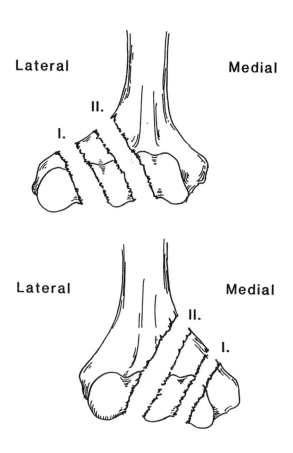

Lateral   Medial

Lateral   Medial

CAPITELLUM FRACTURES

(Bryan and Morrey Classification)

I. CAPITELLUM FRACTURE THAT INVOLVES THE MAJORITY OF THE OSSEOUS PORTION AND MAY EXTEND INTO ADJACENT TROCHLEA

II. SLICE FRACTURE OF THE CAPITELLUM WITH VARIABLE AMOUNT OF ARTICULAR CARTILAGE AND MINIMAL SUBCHONDRAL BONE

III. COMMINUTED OR COMPRESSION FRACTURE

Type I is the most common capitellum fracture.

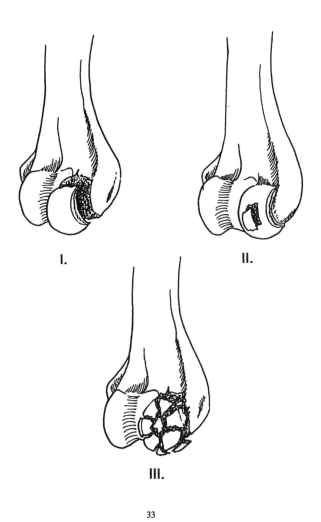

I.

II.

III.

INTERCONDYLAR FRACTURES OF THE HUMERUS

(Riseborough and Radin Classification)

I. NO DISPLACEMENT OF THE FRAGMENTS

II. T-SHAPED FRACTURE WITH THE TROCHLEAR AND CAPITELLAR FRAGMENTS SEPARATED BUT NOT APPRECIABLY ROTATED IN THE FRONTAL PLANE

III. T-SHAPED FRACTURE WITH SEPARATION OF THE FRAGMENTS AND SIGNIFICANT ROTARY DEFORMITY

IV. T-SHAPED INTERCONDYLAR FRACTURES WITH SEVERE COMMINUTION OF THE ARTICULAR SURFACE AND WIDE SEPARATION OF THE HUMERUS CONDYLES

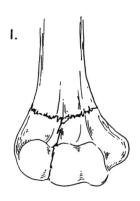

I.

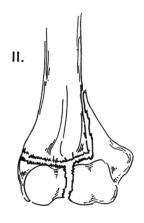

II.

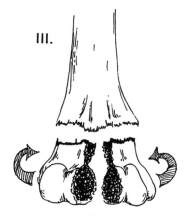

III.

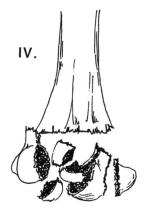

IV.

TRANSCONDYLAR FRACTURES OF THE HUMERUS

(Ashurst Classification)

I.   POSTERIOR DISPLACEMENT

II. ANTERIOR DISPLACEMENT

TRANSCONDYLAR FRACTURES are intercapsular fractures through the condyles. Displacement of the dicondylar fragment is usually posterior.

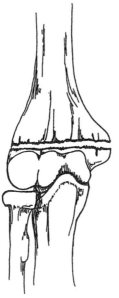

Transcondylar

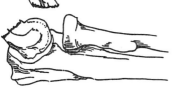

I. Posterior

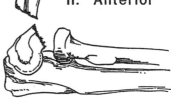

II. Anterior

SUPRACONDYLAR FRACTURES OF THE HUMERUS

(Modified Kocher Classification)

I.   EXTENSION TYPE

II.   FLEXION TYPE

SUPRACONDYLAR EXTENSION FRACTURES are more common than the FLEXION TYPE and approximately 50 percent are completely displaced.

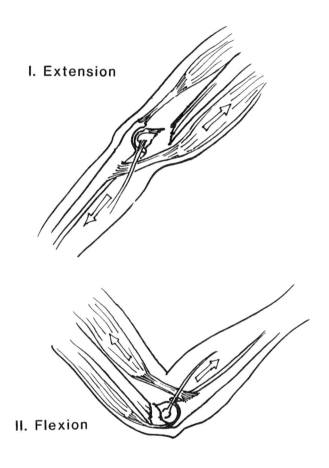

I. Extension

II. Flexion

FRACTURES OF THE PROXIMAL HUMERUS

(Neer Classification)

I. ONE-PART OR MINIMALLY DISPLACED FRACTURE WHERE NO SEGMENTS ARE DISPLACED BY 1.0 CM OR ANGULATED BY 45 DEGREES

II. TWO-PART FRACTURE WHERE ONE SEGMENT IS SIGNIFICANTLY DISPLACED BY 1.0 CM OR 45 DEGREES

III. THREE-PART FRACTURE WHERE TWO SEGMENTS ARE SIGNIFICANTLY DISPLACED BY 1.0 CM OR 45 DEGREES

IV. FOUR-PART FRACTURE WHERE ALL FOUR MAJOR SEGMENTS ARE DISPLACED BY 1.0 CM OR 45 DEGREES

V. FRACTURE DISLOCATION

Classification based on four fracture segments: (1) the articular segment, (2) the greater tuberosity, (3) the lesser tuberosity, and (4) the humeral shaft.

Classification describes only displaced segments which are defined as 1.0 cm displacement or 45 degree angulation.

Multiple fracture configurations are possible.

80 percent of PROXIMAL HUMERAL FRACTURES are minimally displaced.

40

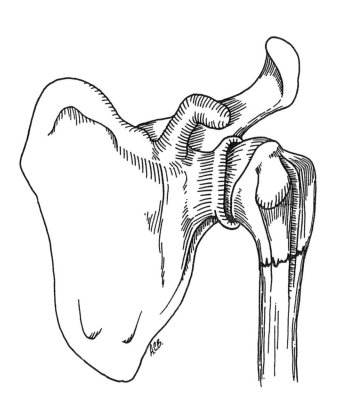

FRACTURES OF THE PROXIMAL HUMERUS

(Neer Classification)

I.   ONE-PART OR MINIMALLY DISPLACED FRACTURE WHERE NO SEGMENTS ARE DISPLACED BY 1.0 CM OR ANGULATED BY 45 DEGREES

II.   TWO-PART FRACTURE WHERE ONE SEGMENT IS SIGNIFICANTLY DISPLACED BY 1.0 CM OR 45 DEGREES

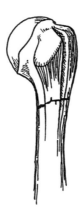

One Part Fracture

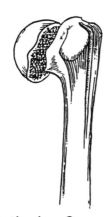

Two Part

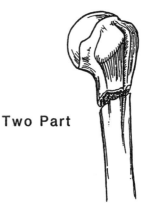

**Articular Segment
Fracture**

**Humeral Shaft
Fracture**

FRACTURES OF THE PROXIMAL HUMERUS

(Neer Classification)

I. ONE-PART OR MINIMALLY DISPLACED FRACTURE WHERE NO SEGMENTS ARE DISPLACED BY 1.0 CM OR ANGULATED BY 45 DEGREES

II. TWO-PART FRACTURE WHERE ONE SEGMENT IS SIGNIFICANTLY DISPLACED BY 1.0 CM OR 45 DEGREES

III. THREE-PART FRACTURE WHERE TWO SEGMENTS ARE SIGNIFICANTLY DISPLACED BY 1.0 CM OR 45 DEGREES

IV. FOUR-PART FRACTURE WHERE ALL FOUR MAJOR SEGMENTS ARE DISPLACED BY 1.0 CM OR 45 DEGREES

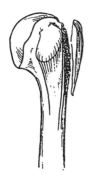

**Two Part
Greater Tuberosity
Fracture**

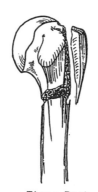

**Three Part
Greater Tuberosity
and Shaft Fracture**

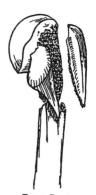

Four Part

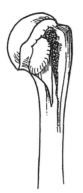

**Two Part
Lesser Tuberosity
Fracture**

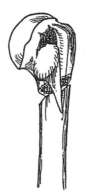

**Three Part
Lesser Tuberosity
and Shaft Fracture**

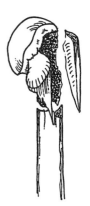

Four Part

45

FRACTURES OF THE PROXIMAL HUMERUS

(Neer Classification)

V.   FRACTURE DISLOCATION

Fracture dislocations may be ANTERIOR or POSTERIOR and are also based on the four fracture segment classification.

Classification describes only displaced segments by 1.0 cm or 45 degree angulation.

Anterior Fracture Dislocations

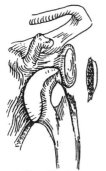

Two Part

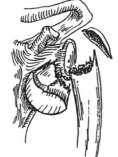

Three Part

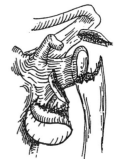

Four Part

Posterior Fracture Dislocations

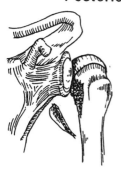

Two Part

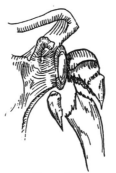

Three Part

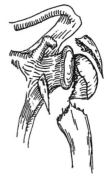

Four Part

FRACTURES OF THE CLAVICLE

(Anatomic Location)

I.   INNER-THIRD - 5%[a]

II. MID-THIRD - 80%

III. DISTAL-THIRD OR INTERLIGAMENTOUS - 15%

DISTAL CLAVICLE FRACTURES are further subdivided on the next page.

[a] *Percentages indicate the frequency of fracture occurrence.*

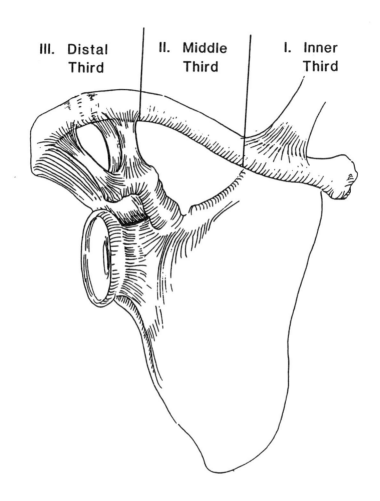

III. Distal
Third

II. Middle
Third

I. Inner
Third

FRACTURES OF THE DISTAL CLAVICLE

(Neer Classification)

I.   INTACT LIGAMENTS WITHOUT SIGNIFICANT DISPLACEMENT

II. DISPLACED INTERLIGAMENTOUS FRACTURE WHERE CORACOCLAVICULAR LIGAMENTS ARE DETACHED FROM THE MEDIAL SEGMENT AND TRAPEZOID LIGAMENTS REMAIN ATTACHED TO THE DISTAL SEGMENT

III. ARTICULAR SURFACE FRACTURES

50

I.

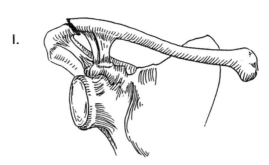

II.

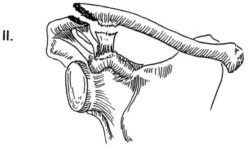

III.

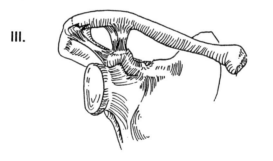

FRACTURES OF THE SCAPULA

(Anatomic Location)

I.   NECK

II. ACROMIUM PROCESS

III. COROCOID PROCESS

IV. BODY

V.   GLENOID RIM OR ARTICULAR SURFACE

VI. SPINOUS PROCESS

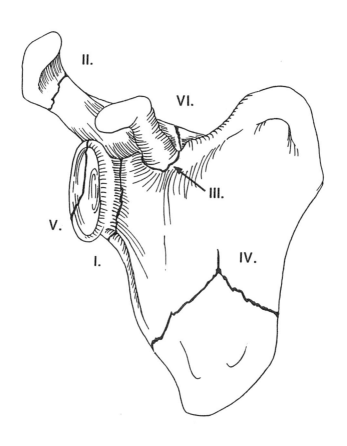

GLENOID FRACTURES

(Ideberg Classification)

I.   FRACTURE OF THE ANTERIOR GLENOID MARGIN; ASSOCIATED WITH
      GLENOHUMERAL FRACTURE DISLOCATION

II.   TRANSVERSE OR OBLIQUE FRACTURE THROUGH THE GLENOID
      FOSSA; MAY BE ASSOCIATED WITH INFERIOR HUMERAL HEAD
      SUBLUXATION OR DISLOCATION

III. OBLIQUE GLENOID FRACTURE THAT COURSES CEPHALAD TO THE
      MID PORTION OF THE SCAPULA

IV.   HORIZONTAL FRACTURE THROUGH THE SCAPULA INVOLVING THE
      GLENOID FOSSA, NECK, AND BODY

V.   HORIZONTAL FRACTURE COMBINED WITH TRANSVERSE COMPONENT
      INVOLVING THE ENTIRE SCAPULAR NECK OR JUST THE
      INFERIOR PORTION

Type I GLENOID FRACTURES are the most common.

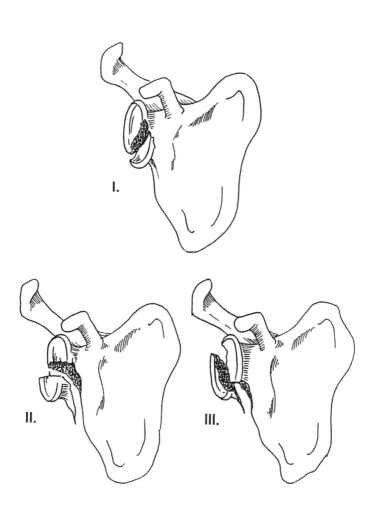

I.

II.

III.

GLENOID FRACTURES

(Ideberg Classification)

IV.   HORIZONTAL FRACTURE THROUGH THE SCAPULA INVOLVING THE GLENOID FOSSA, NECK, AND BODY

V.   HORIZONTAL FRACTURE COMBINED WITH TRANSVERSE COMPONENT INVOLVING THE ENTIRE SCAPULAR NECK OR JUST THE INFERIOR PORTION

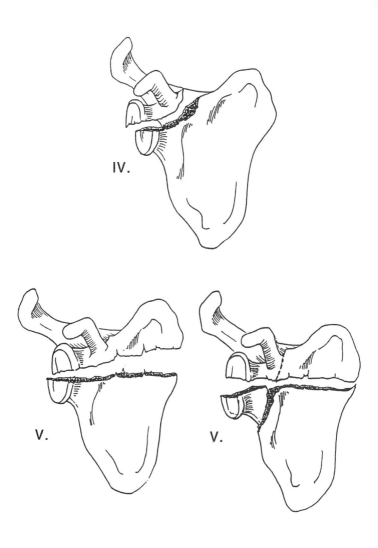

IV.

V.

V.

SPINE

CLASSIFICATION OF CERVICAL SPINE INJURIES

(Harris Classification)

I.   FLEXION

    A.   ANTERIOR SUBLUXATION

    B.   BILATERAL INTERFACETAL DISLOCATION

    C.   SIMPLE WEDGE (COMPRESSION) FRACTURE

    D.   CLAY-SHOVELER (COAL-SHOVELER) FRACTURE

    E.   FLEXION TEARDROP FRACTURE

II. FLEXION-ROTATION: UNILATERAL INTERFACETAL DISLOCATION

III. EXTENSION-ROTATION: PILLAR FRACTURE

IV. VERTICAL COMPRESSION

    A.   JEFFERSON BURST FRACTURE OF ATLAS

    B.   BURST FRACTURE

V.   HYPEREXTENSION

    A.   HYPEREXTENSION DISLOCATION

    B.   AVULSION FRACTURE OF ANTERIOR ARCH OF THE ATLAS

    C.   EXTENSION TEARDROP FRACTURE OF THE AXIS

    D.   FRACTURE OF THE POSTERIOR ARCH OF THE ATLAS

    E.   LAMINAR FRACTURE

    F.   TRAUMATIC SPONDYLOLISTHESIS (HANGMAN'S FRACTURE)

    G.   HYPEREXTENSION FRACTURE DISLOCATION

VI. LATERAL FLEXION: UNCINATE PROCESS FRACTURE

VII. DIVERSE, OR IMPRECISELY UNDERSTOOD, MECHANISMS

    A.   ATLANTA-OCCIPITAL DISASSOCIATION

    B.   ODONTOID FRACTURES

60

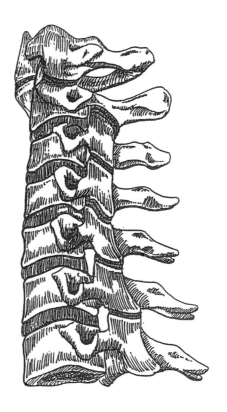

CLASSIFICATION OF CERVICAL SPINE INJURIES

(Harris Classification)

I.   FLEXION

   A.   ANTERIOR SUBLUXATION

   B.   BILATERAL INTERFACETAL DISLOCATION

   C.   SIMPLE WEDGE (COMPRESSION) FRACTURE

   D.   CLAY-SHOVELER (COAL-SHOVELER) FRACTURE

   E.   FLEXION TEARDROP FRACTURE

   Additional descriptions of CLAY-SHOVELER FRACTURE in the EPONYM SECTION.

A.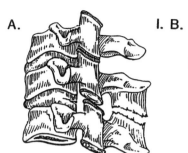

I. B.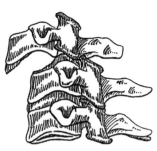

C.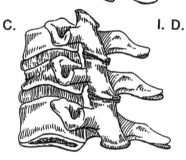

I. D.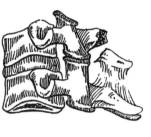

E.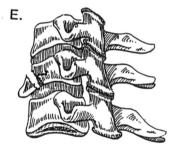

63

CLASSIFICATION OF CERVICAL SPINE INJURIES

(Harris Classification)

II.   FLEXION-ROTATION: UNILATERAL INTERFACETAL DISLOCATION

III.   EXTENSION-ROTATION: PILLAR FRACTURE

II.

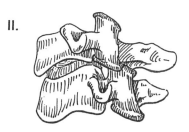

III.

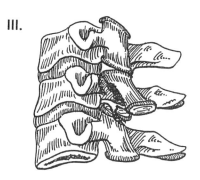

CLASSIFICATION OF CERVICAL SPINE INJURIES

(Harris Classification)

IV.   VERTICAL COMPRESSION

    A.   JEFFERSON BURST FRACTURE OF ATLAS

    B.   BURST FRACTURE

IV. A.

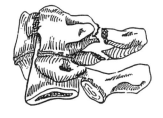 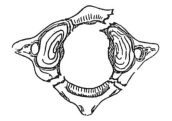

Lateral View   Axial View

IV. B.

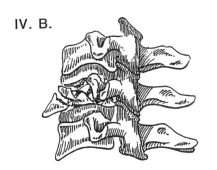

CLASSIFICATION OF CERVICAL SPINE INJURIES

(Harris Classification)

V. HYPEREXTENSION

    A.   HYPEREXTENSION DISLOCATION

    B.   AVULSION FRACTURE OF ANTERIOR ARCH OF THE ATLAS

    C.   EXTENSION TEARDROP FRACTURE OF THE AXIS

    D.   FRACTURE OF THE POSTERIOR ARCH OF THE ATLAS

    E.   LAMINAR FRACTURE

    F.   TRAUMATIC SPONDYLOLISTHESIS (HANGMAN'S FRACTURE)

    G.   HYPERXTENSION FRACTURE DISLOCATION

V. A.

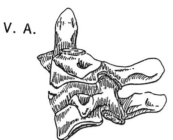

V. B.

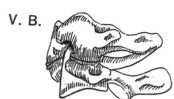

V. C.

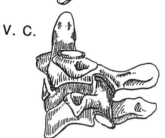

V. D.

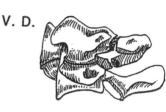

V. E.

V. F.

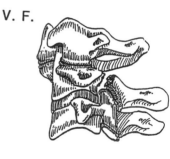

V. G.

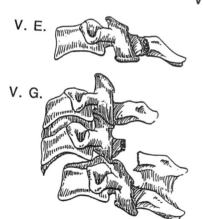

CLASSIFICATION OF CERVICAL SPINE INJURIES

(Harris Classification)

VI.   LATERAL FLEXION: UNCINATE PROCESS FRACTURE

VII.   DIVERSE, OR IMPRECISELY UNDERSTOOD, MECHANISMS

    A.   ATLANTA-OCCIPITAL DISASSOCIATION

    B.   ODONTOID FRACTURES

ODONTOID FRACTURE classification is located on the next page.

VI.

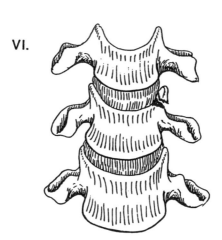

VII. A.

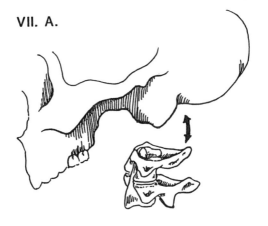

FRACTURES OF THE ODONTOID PROCESS

(Anderson and D'Alonzo Classification)

I. OBLIQUE FRACTURE THROUGH THE SUPERIOR PART OF THE ODONTOID

II. FRACTURE AT THE JUNCTION OF THE ODONTOID PROCESS AND THE AXIS

III. FRACTURE EXTENDS INTO THE BODY OF THE AXIS

ODONTOID FRACTURES may be further classified as *DISPLACED* or *NONDISPLACED.*

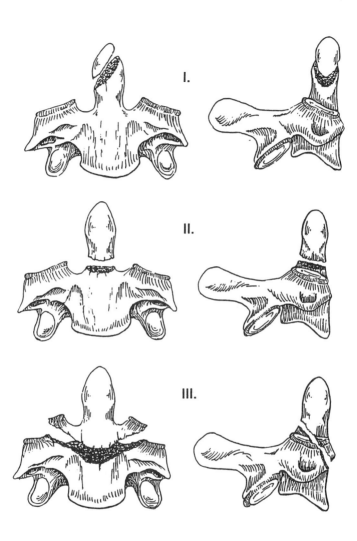

I.

II.

III.

THORACOLUMBAR SPINAL INJURY CLASSIFICATION

(Denis Classification)

I.   MINOR SPINAL INJURIES

    A.   ARTICULAR PROCESS FRACTURE

    B.   TRANSVERSE PROCESS FRACTURE

    C.   SPINOUS PROCESS FRACTURE

    D.   PARS INTERARTICULARIS FRACTURE

II. MAJOR SPINAL INJURIES

    A.   COMPRESSION FRACTURE

    B.   BURST FRACTURES

    C.   FRACTURE DISLOCATIONS

    D.   SEAT-BELT TYPE SPINAL INJURIES

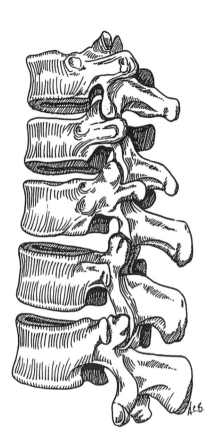

THORACOLUMBAR SPINAL INJURY CLASSIFICATION

(Denis Classification)

I.   MINOR SPINAL INJURIES

    A.   TRANSVERSE PROCESS FRACTURE

    B.   ARTICULAR PROCESS FRACTURE

    C.   SPINOUS PROCESS FRACTURE

    D.   PARS INTERARTICULARIS FRACTURE

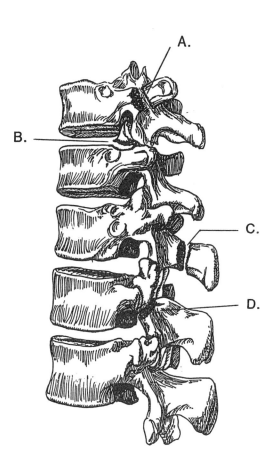

A.

B.

C.

D.

THORACOLUMBAR SPINAL INJURY CLASSIFICATION

(Denis Classification)

II.   MAJOR SPINAL INJURIES

    A.   COMPRESSION FRACTURE

    B.   BURST FRACTURES

BURST FRACTURES disrupt middle spinal segment and retropulse bone fragments toward the spinal canal.

II. A.

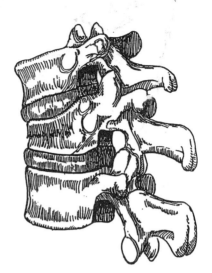

II. B.

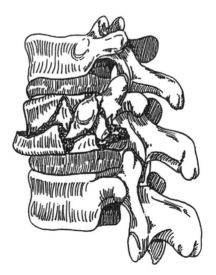

THORACOLUMBAR SPINAL INJURY CLASSIFICATION

(Denis Classification)

II.   MAJOR SPINAL INJURIES

      C.   FRACTURE DISLOCATIONS

      D.   SEAT-BELT TYPE SPINAL INJURIES

SEAT-BELT TYPE SPINAL INJURIES may be through bone, ligaments or a combination. Mechanism of injury is usually a flexion distraction type force.

II. C.

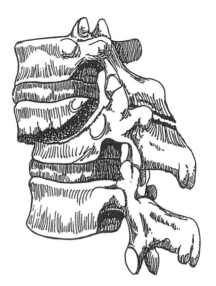

II. D.

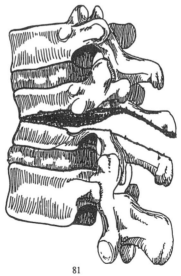

PELVIS
and
ACETABULUM

CLASSIFICATION OF PELVIC DISRUPTION

(Tile Classification)

TYPE A.   STABLE

    A1.   FRACTURES OF THE PELVIS NOT INVOLVING THE RING

    A2.   STABLE, MINIMALLY DISPLACED FRACTURES OF THE RING

TYPE B.   ROTATIONALLY UNSTABLE, VERTICALLY STABLE

    B1.   OPEN BOOK

    B2.   LATERAL COMPRESSION: IPSILATERAL

    B3.   LATERAL COMPRESSION: CONTRALATERAL (BUCKET HANDLE)

TYPE C.   ROTATIONALLY AND VERTICALLY UNSTABLE

    C1.   UNILATERAL

    C2.   BILATERAL

    C3.   ASSOCIATED WITH ACETABULAR FRACTURE

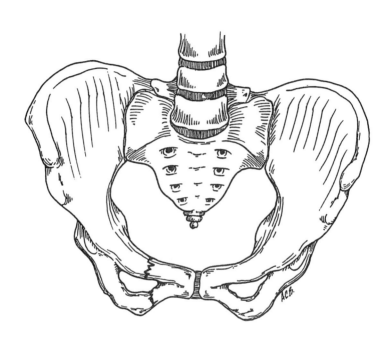

CLASSIFICATION OF PELVIC DISRUPTION

(Tile Classification)

TYPE A.   STABLE

    A1.   FRACTURES OF THE PELVIS NOT INVOLVING THE RING

    A2.   STABLE, MINIMALLY DISPLACED FRACTURES OF THE RING

A. 1.

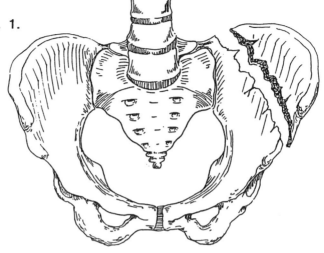

A. 2.

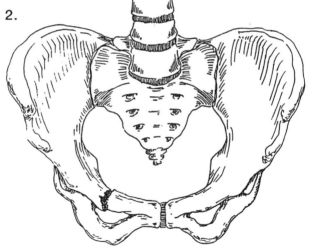

CLASSIFICATION OF PELVIC DISRUPTION

(Tile Classification)

TYPE B.   ROTATIONALLY UNSTABLE, VERTICALLY STABLE

B1.   OPEN BOOK

B2.   LATERAL COMPRESSION: IPSILATERAL

B. 1.

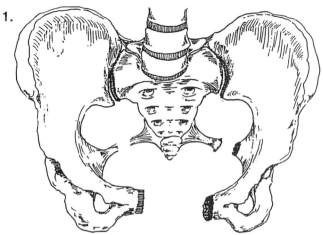

B. 2.

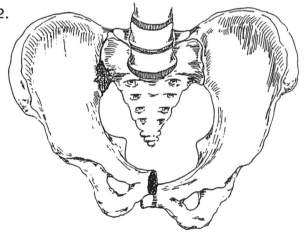

CLASSIFICATION OF PELVIC DISRUPTION

(Tile Classification)

TYPE B.   ROTATIONALLY UNSTABLE, VERTICALLY STABLE

   B3.   LATERAL COMPRESSION: CONTRALATERAL (BUCKET HANDLE)

B. 3.

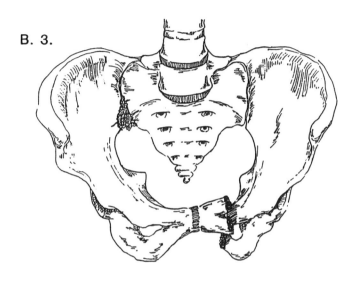

CLASSIFICATION OF PELVIC DISRUPTION

(Tile Classification)

TYPE C.   ROTATIONALLY AND VERTICALLY UNSTABLE

    C1.   UNILATERAL

    C2.   BILATERAL

    C3.   ASSOCIATED WITH ACETABULAR FRACTURE

C. 1.

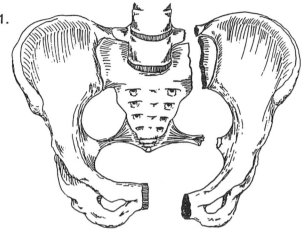

C. 2.

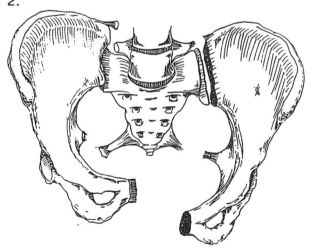

CLASSIFICATION OF ACETABULUM FRACTURES

(Tile Classification)

UNDISPLACED

DISPLACED

TYPE I.   POSTERIOR TYPES WITH OR WITHOUT POSTERIOR DISLOCATION

    A.   POSTERIOR COLUMN

    B.   POSTERIOR WALL

        1.   ASSOCIATED WITH POSTERIOR COLUMN

        2.   ASSOCIATED WITH TRANSVERSE FRACTURES

TYPE II.   ANTERIOR TYPES WITH OR WITHOUT ANTERIOR DISLOCATIONS

    A.   ANTERIOR COLUMN

    B.   ANTERIOR WALL

    C.   ASSOCIATED WITH ANTERIOR WALL, ANTERIOR COLUMN, AND/OR TRANSVERSE FRACTURES

TYPE III.   TRANSVERSE TYPES WITH OR WITHOUT CENTRAL DISLOCATION

    A.   PURE TRANSVERSE

    B.   T-FRACTURES

    C.   ASSOCIATED TRANSVERSE AND ACETABULAR WALL FRACTURES

    D.   DOUBLE COLUMN FRACTURES

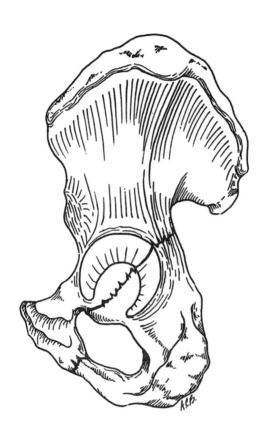

CLASSIFICATION OF ACETABULUM FRACTURES

(Tile Classification)

DISPLACED

TYPE I.   POSTERIOR TYPES WITH OR WITHOUT POSTERIOR DISLOCATION

    A.   POSTERIOR COLUMN

    B.   POSTERIOR WALL

        1.   ASSOCIATED WITH POSTERIOR COLUMN

        2.   ASSOCIATED WITH TRANSVERSE FRACTURES

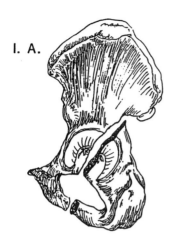
I. A.

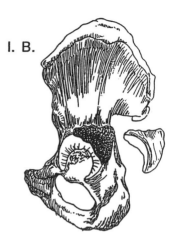
I. B.

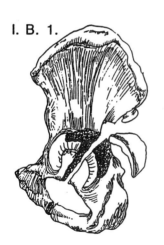
I. B. 1.

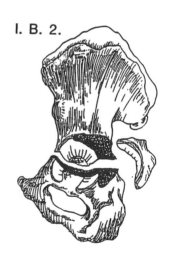
I. B. 2.

97

CLASSIFICATION OF ACETABULUM FRACTURES

(Tile Classification)

DISPLACED

TYPE II.   ANTERIOR TYPES WITH OR WITHOUT ANTERIOR DISLOCATIONS

    A.   ANTERIOR COLUMN

    B.   ANTERIOR WALL

    C.   ASSOCIATED WITH ANTERIOR WALL, ANTERIOR COLUMN, AND/OR TRANSVERSE FRACTURES

II. A.

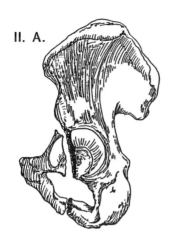

II. B.

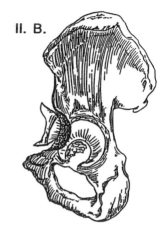

II. C.

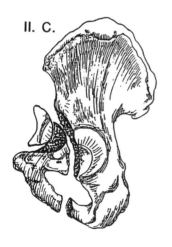

II. C.

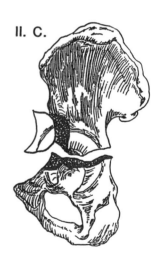

CLASSIFICATION OF ACETABULUM FRACTURES

(Tile Classification)

DISPLACED

TYPE III. TRANSVERSE TYPES WITH OR WITHOUT CENTRAL DISLOCATION

    A. PURE TRANSVERSE

    B. T-FRACTURES

    C. ASSOCIATED TRANSVERSE AND ACETABULAR WALL FRACTURES

    D. DOUBLE COLUMN FRACTURES

III. A.

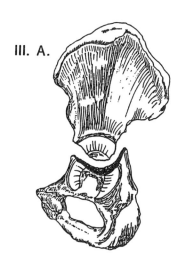

III. B.

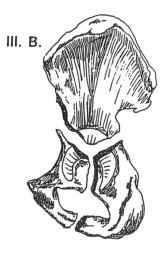

III. C.

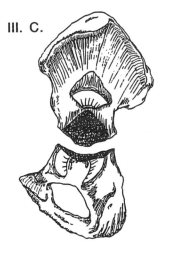

III. D.

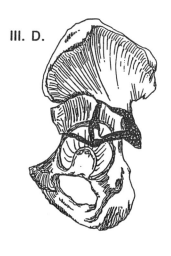

SACRAL FRACTURE CLASSIFICATION

(Denis Classification)

I.   FRACTURE THROUGH SACRAL ALA WITHOUT DAMAGE TO THE CENTRAL CANAL OR SACRAL FORAMINA

II.   FRACTURE INVOLVING THE SACRAL FORAMINA BUT SPARING THE CENTRAL CANAL. FRACTURE MAY ALSO INVOLVE THE ALAR ZONE

III.   FRACTURE INVOLVING THE CENTRAL SACRAL CANAL. FRACTURE MAY ALSO INVOLVE FORAMINA AND ALAR ZONES

Zone II fractures are frequently associated with sciatica and nerve root injury.

Zone III fractures are frequently associated with loss of sphincter function and saddle anesthesia.

I.   II.   III.

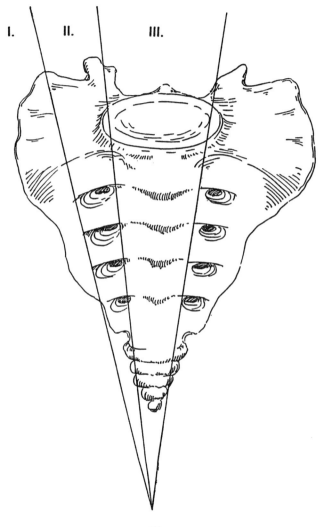

103

LOWER EXTREMITY

CLASSIFICATION OF HIP FRACTURES

(Anatomic Classification)

I.   FEMORAL NECK - INTRACAPSULAR FRACTURES
       (Garden Classification)

II.   INTERTROCHANTERIC - EXTRACAPSULAR FRACTURE
       (Kyle Classification)

III.   SUBTROCHANTERIC
       (Seinsheimer Classification)

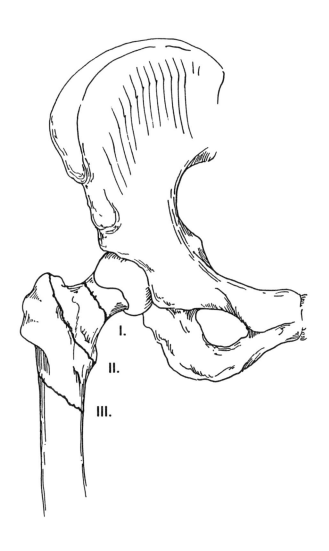

I.

II.

III.

POSTERIOR HIP DISLOCATIONS
ASSOCIATED WITH FEMORAL HEAD FRACTURES

(Pipkin Classification)

I.   POSTERIOR DISLOCATION WITH FRACTURE OF THE FEMORAL HEAD CAUDAD TO THE FOVEA CENTRALIS

II.   POSTERIOR DISLOCATION WITH FRACTURE OF THE FEMORAL HEAD CEPHALAD TO THE FOVEA CENTRALIS

III.   TYPE I OR II WITH FEMORAL NECK FRACTURE

IV.   TYPE I, II, OR III WITH ASSOCIATED ACETABULUM FRACTURE

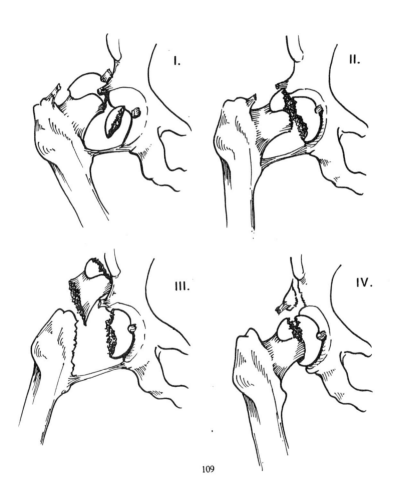

FRACTURES OF THE FEMORAL NECK

(Garden Classification)

I.   INCOMPLETE OR IMPACTED FRACTURE

II.   COMPLETE FRACTURE WITHOUT DISPLACEMENT

III. COMPLETE FRACTURE WITH PARTIAL DISPLACEMENT
      (HIP CAPSULE USUALLY PARTIALLY INTACT)

IV.   COMPLETE FRACTURE WITH FULL DISPLACEMENT
      (HIP CAPSULE USUALLY COMPLETELY DISRUPTED)

Greater fracture displacement increases the incidence of avascular necrosis.

Type I femoral neck fractures may present with coxa valgus, while type III fractures demonstrate coxa varus.

110

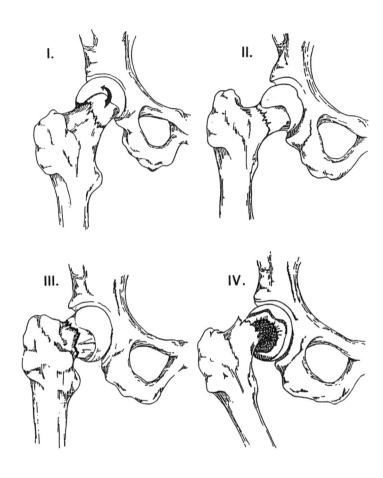

I.

II.

III.

IV.

111

INTERTROCHANTERIC HIP FRACTURES

(Kyle Classification)

I. NONDISPLACED STABLE INTERTROCHANTERIC FRACTURE WITHOUT COMMINUTION

II. DISPLACED STABLE INTERTROCHANTERIC FRACTURE WITH MINIMAL COMMINUTION

III. DISPLACED UNSTABLE INTERTROCHANTERIC FRACTURE WITH EXTENSIVE POSTERIOR MEDIAL COMMINUTION

IV. DISPLACED UNSTABLE INTERTROCHANTERIC FRACTURE WITH EXTENSIVE POSTERIOR MEDIAL COMMINUTION AND A SUBTROCHANTERIC COMPONENT

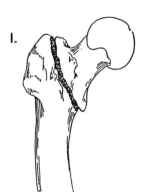

I.

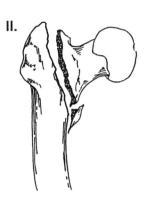

II.

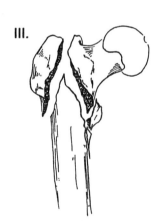

III.

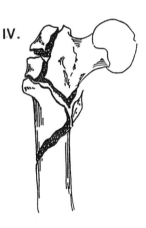

IV.

113

SUBTROCHANTERIC FRACTURES OF THE FEMUR

(Seinsheimer Classification)

I.   NONDISPLACED FRACTURE WITH LESS THAN 2 MM OF DISPLACEMENT

II.   TWO-PART FRACTURES

    IIA.   TWO-PART TRANSVERSE FEMORAL FRACTURE

    IIB.   TWO-PART SPIRAL FRACTURE WITH LESSER TROCHANTER ATTACHED TO PROXIMAL FRAGMENT

    IIC.   TWO-PART SPIRAL FRACTURE WITH LESSER TROCHANTER ATTACHED TO DISTAL FRAGMENT

III.   THREE-PART FRACTURES

    IIIA.   THREE-PART SPIRAL FRACTURE IN WHICH THE LESSER TROCHANTER IS PART OF THE THIRD FRAGMENT

    IIIB.   THREE-PART SPIRAL FRACTURE IN WHICH THE THIRD PART IS A BUTTERFLY FRAGMENT

IV.   COMMINUTED FRACTURE WITH FOUR OR MORE FRAGMENTS

V.   SUBTROCHANTERIC INTERTROCHANTERIC FRACTURE, ANY SUBTROCHANTERIC FRACTURE WITH EXTENSION THROUGH THE GREATER TROCHANTER

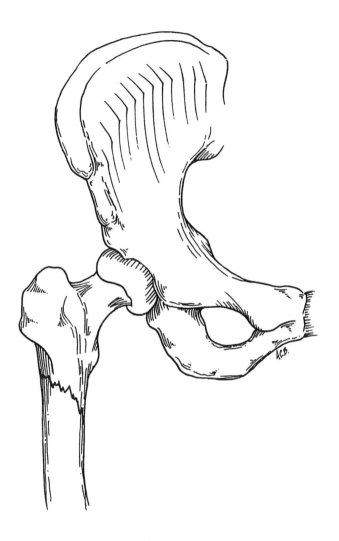

115

SUBTROCHANTERIC FRACTURES OF THE FEMUR

(Seinsheimer Classification)

I. NONDISPLACED FRACTURE WITH LESS THAN 2 MM OF DISPLACEMENT

II. TWO-PART FRACTURES

    IIA. TWO-PART TRANSVERSE FEMORAL FRACTURE

    IIB. TWO-PART SPIRAL FRACTURE WITH LESSER TROCHANTER ATTACHED TO PROXIMAL FRAGMENT

    IIC. TWO-PART SPIRAL FRACTURE WITH LESSER TROCHANTER ATTACHED TO DISTAL FRAGMENT

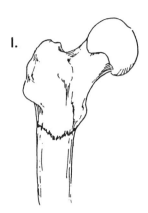

I.

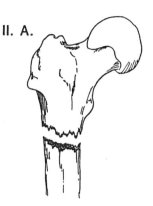

II. A.

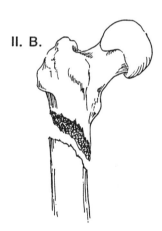

II. B.

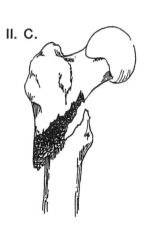

II. C.

SUBTROCHANTERIC FRACTURES OF THE FEMUR

(Seinsheimer Classification)

III. THREE-PART FRACTURES

    IIIA. THREE-PART SPIRAL FRACTURE IN WHICH THE LESSER TROCHANTER IS PART OF THE THIRD FRAGMENT

    IIIB. THREE-PART SPIRAL FRACTURE IN WHICH THE THIRD PART IS A BUTTERFLY FRAGMENT

IV. COMMINUTED FRACTURE WITH FOUR OR MORE FRAGMENTS

V. SUBTROCHANTERIC - INTERTROCHANTERIC FRACTURE

118

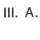

III. A.

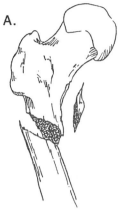

III. B.

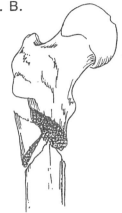

IV.

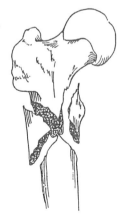

V.

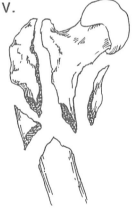

119

FEMORAL SHAFT FRACTURES

(Winquist Classification of Comminution)

I. FEMORAL SHAFT FRACTURE WITH VERY SMALL BUTTERFLY FRAGMENT (25% OR LESS OF THE WIDTH OF THE BONE)

II. COMMINUTED FEMORAL SHAFT FRACTURE WITH BUTTERFLY FRAGMENT 50% OR LESS OF THE WIDTH OF THE BONE

III. COMMINUTED FRACTURE WITH LARGE BUTTERFLY SEGMENT GREATER THAN 50% OF THE WIDTH OF THE BONE

IV. SEVERE COMMINUTION OF AN ENTIRE SEGMENT OF BONE

V. FEMORAL SHAFT FRACTURE WITH SEGMENTAL BONE LOSS

Increasing comminution decreases inherent stability to rotation, shortening, and angulation.

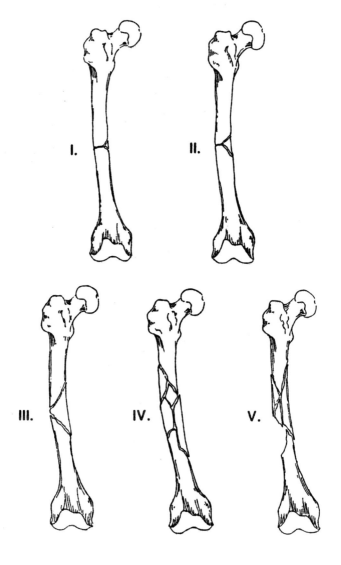

I.

II.

III.

IV.

V.

SUPRACONDYLAR FEMORAL FRACTURES

(AO Classification)

A. EXTRA-ARTICULAR

    A1. AVULSION OF THE MEDIAL OR LATERAL EPICONDYLE

    A2. SIMPLE SUPRACONDYLAR

    A3. COMMINUTED SUPRACONDYLAR

B. UNICONDYLAR

    B1. MEDIAL OR LATERAL CONDYLE

    B2. CONDYLE FRACTURE WITH EXTENSION PROXIMALLY INTO FEMORAL SHAFT

    B3. POSTERIOR TANGENTIAL FRACTURE OF ONE OR BOTH CONDYLES

C. BICONDYLAR

    C1. INTERCONDYLAR

    C2. INTERCONDYLAR WITH A COMMINUTED SUPRACONDYLAR COMPONENT

    C3. SEVERLY COMMINUTED BICONDYLAR FRACTURE

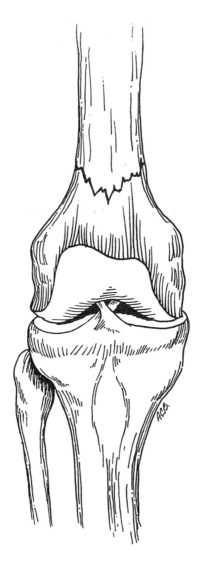

123

SUPRACONDYLAR FEMORAL FRACTURES

(AO Classification)

A. EXTRA-ARTICULAR

A1. AVULSION OF THE MEDIAL OR LATERAL EPICONDYLE

A2. SIMPLE SUPRACONDYLAR

A3. COMMINUTED SUPRACONDYLAR

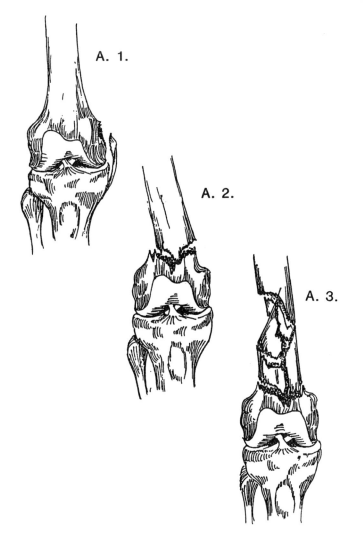

A. 1.

A. 2.

A. 3.

125

SUPRACONDYLAR FEMORAL FRACTURES

(AO Classification)

B.   UNICONDYLAR

   B1.   MEDIAL OR LATERAL CONDYLE

   B2.   CONDYLE FRACTURE WITH EXTENSION PROXIMALLY INTO
          FEMORAL SHAFT

   B3.   POSTERIOR TANGENTIAL FRACTURE OF ONE OR BOTH
          CONDYLES

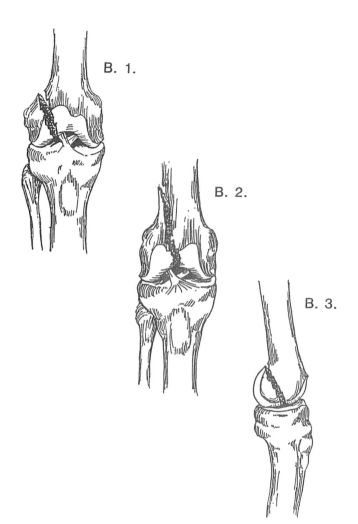

B. 1.

B. 2.

B. 3.

SUPRACONDYLAR FEMORAL FRACTURES

(AO Classification)

C.   BICONDYLAR

   C1.   INTERCONDYLAR

   C2.   INTERCONDYLAR WITH A COMMINUTED SUPRACONDYLAR
            COMPONENT

   C3.   SEVERLY COMMINUTED BICONDYLAR FRACTURE

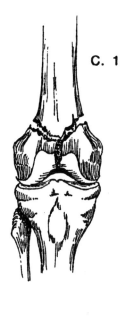

C. 1.

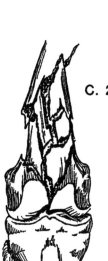

C. 2.

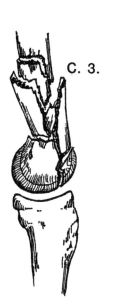

C. 3.

129

PATELLA FRACTURES

(Fracture Configuration Classification)

I.   NONDISPLACED

II.   TRANSVERSE

III.   UPPER OR LOWER POLE

IV.   COMMINUTED

V.   VERTICAL

I.

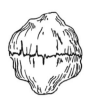

II.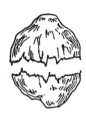

III.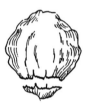

IV.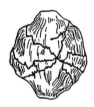

V.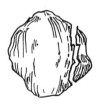

FRACTURES OF THE TIBIAL SPINE

(Meyers Classification)

I.   FRACTURE TILTED UP ONLY ANTERIORLY

II.   ANTERIOR PORTION LIFTED COMPLETELY FROM TIBIA WITH ONLY
      SOME POSTERIOR ATTACHMENT

IIIA. INTERCONDYLAR FRAGMENT NOT IN CONTACT WITH THE TIBIA

IIIB. INTERCONDYLAR FRAGMENT ROTATED

I.

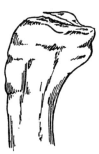
II.

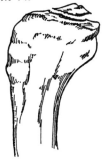
III. A.

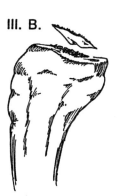
III. B.

FRACTURES OF THE TIBIAL PLATEAU

(Schatzker Classification)

I. CLEAVAGE OR WEDGE TYPE FRACTURES OF THE LATERAL TIBIAL PLATEAU - 24%[a]

II. LATERAL WEDGE FRACTURE WITH ADJACENT DEPRESSION - 26%

III. PURE CENTRAL DEPRESSION WITHOUT AN ASSOCIATED WEDGE FRACTURE - 26%

IV. WEDGE OR DEPRESSION FRACTURES OF THE MEDIAL TIBIAL PLATEAU - 11%

V. BICONDYLAR FRACTURE OF THE TIBIAL PLATEAU - 10%

VI. TIBIAL PLATEAU FRACTURE WITH DISASSOCIATION OF THE METAPHYSIS FROM THE DIAPHYSIS BY A FRACTURE - 3%

[a] *Percentages indicate the frequency of fracture occurrence.*

134

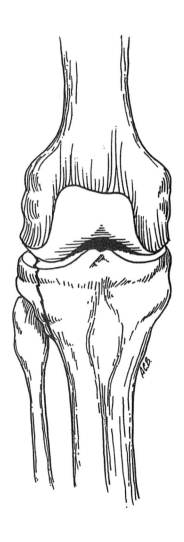

FRACTURES OF THE TIBIAL PLATEAU

(Schatzker Classification)

I.   CLEAVAGE OR WEDGE TYPE FRACTURES OF THE LATERAL TIBIAL
     PLATEAU

II. LATERAL WEDGE FRACTURE WITH ADJACENT DEPRESSION

III. PURE CENTRAL DEPRESSION WITHOUT AN ASSOCIATED WEDGE
     FRACTURE

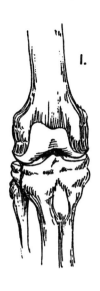

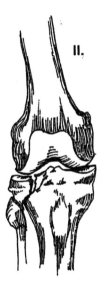

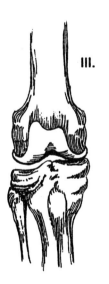

FRACTURES OF THE TIBIAL PLATEAU

(Schatzker Classification)

IV. WEDGE OR DEPRESSION FRACTURES OF THE MEDIAL TIBIAL PLATEAU

V. BICONDYLAR FRACTURE OF THE TIBIAL PLATEAU

VI. TIBIAL PLATEAU FRACTURE WITH DISASSOCIATION OF THE METAPHYSIS FROM THE DIAPHYSIS BY A FRACTURE

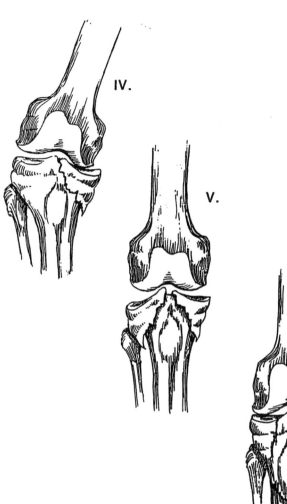

IV.

V.

VI.

139

TIBIAL SHAFT FRACTURES

(Chapman Classification)

A.   TRANSVERSE OR SHORT OBLIQUE

B.   SMALL BUTTERFLY FRAGMENT

C.   LARGE BUTTERFLY FRAGMENT

D.   SEGMENTAL COMMINUTION

E.   SPIRAL

F.   PROMIMAL ONE-FOURTH TRANSVERSE OR OBLIQUE

G.   DISTAL ONE-FOURTH TRANSVERSE OR OBLIQUE

Type A is usually stable; B and C stability depend on the size of the butterfly fragment.

Type D is usually unstable while types E, F and G are stable but difficult to control.

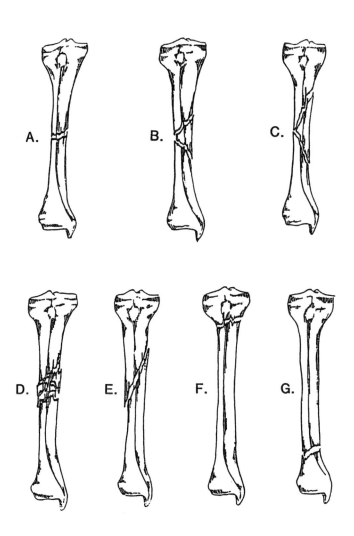

FRACTURES OF THE DISTAL TIBIA
WITH INTRA-ARTICULAR EXTENSION - PILON FRACTURE

(AO Classification)

I. CLEAVAGE FRACTURES OF THE ARTICULAR SURFACE WITHOUT SIGNIFICANT DISPLACEMENT

II. CLEAVAGE FRACTURES OF THE ARTICULAR SURFACE WITH SIGNIFICANT ARTICULAR INCONGRUITY, BUT WITHOUT EXTENSIVE COMMINUTION

III. CLEAVAGE FRACTURES OF THE ARTICULAR SURFACE WITH SIGNIFICANT COMPRESSION, DISPLACEMENT, AND COMMINUTION

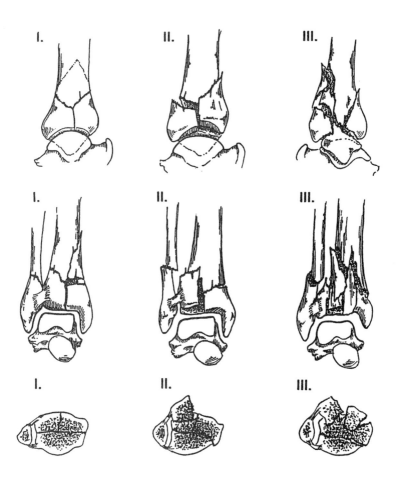

ANKLE FRACTURE CLASSIFICATIONS[a]

(AO Classification)

(Lauge - Hansen Classification)

AO CLASSIFICATION

    A.   TRANSVERSE FIBULA FRACTURE AT OR BELOW JOINT LINE

    B.   SPRAL FIBULA FRACTURE BEGINNING AT JOINT LINE

    C.   OBLIQUE FIBULA FRACTURE ABOVE ANKLE MORTISE

LAUGE - HANSEN CLASSIFICATION

    A.   SUPINATION - EVERSION

    B.   SUPINATION - ADDUCTION

    C.   PRONATION - ABDUCTION

    D.   PRONATION - EVERSION

    E.   PRONATION - DORSIFLEXION

[a] *Two widely used classifications exist for ankle fractures.*

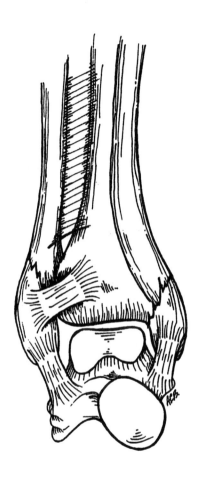

ANKLE FRACTURE CLASSIFICATIONS

(Danis-Weber Classification)

A.   TRANSVERSE FIBULA FRACTURE AT OR BELOW THE JOINT LINE WITH
      POSSIBLE SHEAR FRACTURE OF THE MEDIAL MALLEOLUS.
      TIBIOFIBULAR SYNDESMOSIS INTACT.

B.   SPIRAL FIBULA FRACTURE BEGINNING AT THE JOINT LINE WITH
      ASSOCIATED MEDIAL INJURY. ANTERIOR SYNDESMOSIS MAY
      BE TORN BUT POSTERIOR IS USUALLY INTACT. OVERALL
      INTEGRITY OF THE TIBIOFIBULAR SYNDESMOSIS IS INTACT.

C1. OBLIQUE FIBULA FRACTURE ABOVE A RUPTURED TIBIOFIBULAR
      LIGAMENT WITH ASSOCIATED MEDIAL INJURY. TIBIOFIBULAR
      SYNDESMOSIS IS ALWAYS DISRUPTED.

C2. OBIQUE FIBULA FRACTURE WELL ABOVE ANKLE MORTISE WITH
      EXTENSIVE TIBIOFIBULAR SYNDESMOSIS DISRUPTION.

This classification emphasizes the fibula fracture.

The more proximal the fibular fracture, the greater the syndesmosis injury and
displacement of the ankle mortise.

146

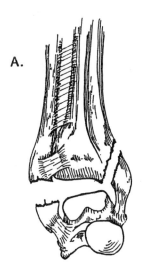

A.

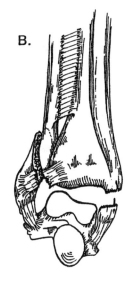

B.

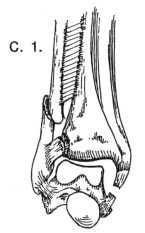

C. 1.

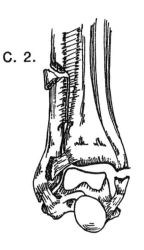

C. 2.

147

ANKLE FRACTURE CLASSIFICATIONS

(Lauge - Hansen Classification)

A. **SUPINATION - EVERSION**

    I.   DISRUPTION OF THE ANTERIOR TIBIOFIBULAR LIGAMENT

    II.   SPIRAL OBLIQUE FRACTURE OF THE DISTAL FIBULA

    III.   DISRUPTION POSTERIOR TIBIOFIBULAR LIGAMENT, MAY FRACTURE POSTERIOR TIBIA

    IV.   MEDIAL MALLEOLUS FRACTURE OR DELTOID LIGAMENT TEAR

B. **SUPINATION - ADDUCTION**

    I.   TRANSVERSE FRACTURE LATERAL MALLEOLUS OR RUPTURE COLLATERAL LIGAMENT

    II.   VERTICAL FRACTURE OF MEDIAL MALLEOLUS

SUPINATION - EVERSION is the most common type.

The Lauge - Hansen Classification is based on mechanism of injury. The first word in the classification refers to the position of the foot (SUPINATION or PRONATION) at the time of injury. The second word refers to the direction of the deforming force.

Each of the four injury categories are subdivided into stages indicating increasing severity of injury. Higher stages indicate more severe injury and worse prognosis.

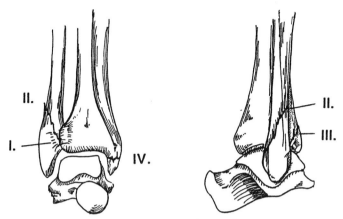

A. Supination Eversion

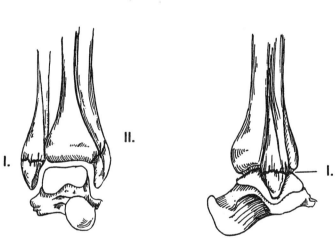

B. Supination Adduction

149

ANKLE FRACTURE CLASSIFICATIONS

(Lauge - Hansen Classification)

C. PRONATION - ABDUCTION

   I.   TRANSVERSE FRACTURE OF THE MEDIAL MALLEOLUS OR DELTOID LIGAMENT RUPTURE

   II. ANTERIOR AND POSTURE TIBIOFIBULAR LIGAMENT RUPTURE WITH OR WITHOUT FRAGMENT OF POSTERIOR MARGIN OF THE TIBIA

   III. SHORT HORIZONTALLY DIRECTED OBLIQUE FIBULA FRACTURE

D. PRONATION - EVERSION

   I.   FRACTURE OF THE MEDIAL MALLEOLUS OR RUPTURE OF THE DELTOID LIGAMENT

   II. TEAR OF THE ANTERIOR TIBIOFIBULAR AND INTEROSSEOUS LIGAMENTS

   III. SPIRAL FRACTURE OF THE FIBULA 7 TO 8 CM PROXIMAL TO THE TIP OF THE LATERAL MALLEOLUS

   IV. FRACTURE OF THE POSTERIOR LIP OF THE TIBIA

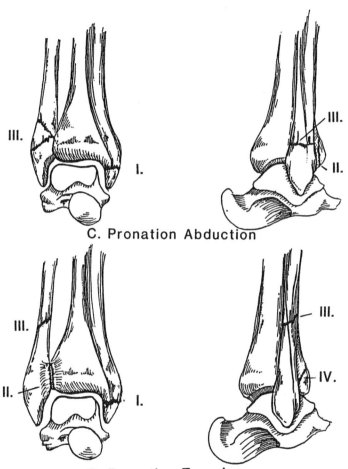

C. Pronation Abduction

D. Pronation Eversion

ANKLE FRACTURE CLASSIFICATIONS

(Lauge - Hansen Classification)

E. PRONATION - DORSIFLEXION

  I.   FRACTURE OF THE MEDIAL MALLEOLUS OR RUPTURE OF THE DELTOID LIGAMENT

  II. ANTERIOR ARTICULAR TIBIA FRACTURE CAUSED BY DORSIFLEXION OF THE TALUS

  III. SUPRAMALLEOLAR FIBULA FRACTURE

  IV. AVULSION FRACTURE OF THE POSTERIOR TIBIA CAUSED BY CONTINUED DORSIFLEXION OF THE TALUS

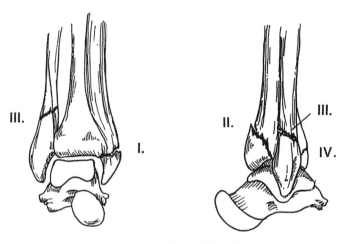

E. Pronation Dorsiflexion

FRACTURES OF THE NECK OF THE TALUS

(Modified Hawkins Classification)

I.   NONDISPLACED VERTICAL FRACTURE

II. DISPLACED FRACTURE WITH SUBLUXATION OR DISLOCATION OF THE
     SUBTALAR JOINT, BUT THE ANKLE MORTISE REMAINS INTACT

III. DISPLACED FRACTURE WITH BOTH SUBTALAR AND TIBIOTALAR
     DISLOCATIONS

IV. DISPLACED FRACTURE WITH DISLOCATION OF THE NECK FRAGMENT,
     WHILE THE BODY REMAINS REDUCED

Rate of avascular necrosis of the talus is related to the degree of fracture displacement.

Type IV fractures are rare.

No muscles or tendons originate or insert on talus.

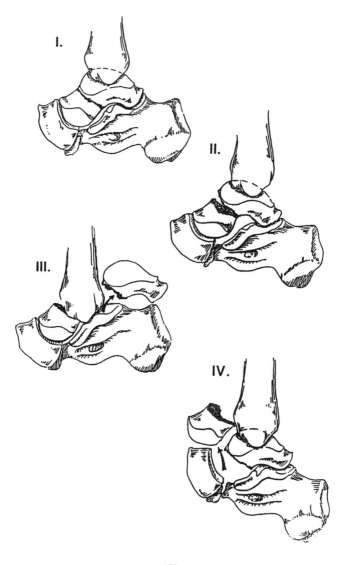

I.

II.

III.

IV.

155

TALAR BODY FRACTURES

(DeLee Classification)

GROUP I.   COMPRESSION OR TRANSCHONDRAL FRACTURES OF THE TALAR DOME; INCLUDES OSTEOCHONDRITIS DISSECANS OF THE TALUS

GROUP II.   CORONAL, SAGGITAL, OR HORIZONTAL SHEARING FRACTURES OF THE ENTIRE TALAR BODY

GROUP III.   POSTERIOR TUBERCLE FRACTURE OF THE TALUS

GROUP IV.   LATERAL PROCESS TALAR FRACTURE

GROUP V.   TALAR BODY CRUSH FRACTURES

Talar body fractures are uncommon and constitute approximately 1 % of all fractures.

156

I.

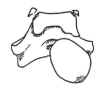

II.

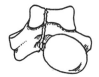
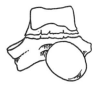

III.

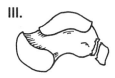

IV.

V.

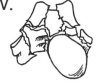

FRACTURES OF THE CALCANEUS

(Essex - Lopresti Classification)

I. EXTRA-ARTICULAR FRACTURES - 25%[a]

    A. ANTERIOR PROCESS - AVULSION OR COMPRESSION

    B. TUBEROSITY

    C. MEDIAL PROCESS

    D. SUSTENACULUM TALI

    E. BODY WITHOUT INVOLVEMENT OF THE SUBTALAR JOINT

II. INTRA-ARTICULAR FRACTURES - 75%

    A. NONDISPLACED

    B. JOINT DEPRESSION

    C. TONGUE TYPE

    D. SEVERELY COMMINUTED

[a] *Percentages indicate the frequency of fracture occurrence.*

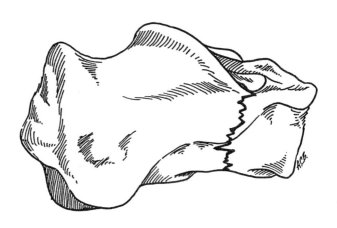

FRACTURES OF THE CALCANEUS

(Essex - Lopresti Classification)

I. EXTRA-ARTICULAR FRACTURES - 25%

    A. ANTERIOR PROCESS - AVULSION OR COMPRESSION

    B. TUBEROSITY

    C. MEDIAL PROCESS

    D. SUSTENACULUM TALI

    E. BODY WITHOUT INVOLVEMENT OF THE SUBTALAR JOINT

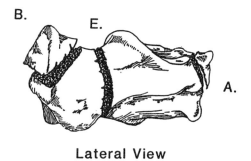

Lateral View

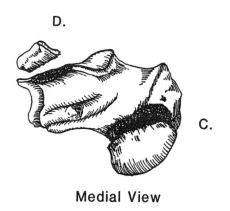

Medial View

FRACTURES OF THE CALCANEUS

(Essex - Lopresti Classification)

II.   INTRA-ARTICULAR FRACTURES - 75%

  A.   NONDISPLACED

  B.   JOINT DEPRESSION

  C.   TONGUE TYPE

  D.   SEVERELY COMMINUTED

INTRA-ARTICULAR CALCANEUS FRACTURES are frequently associated with other injuries, including ipsilateral lower extremity injuries and thoracolumbar spine fractures.

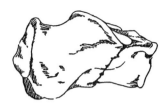

A.

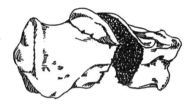

B.

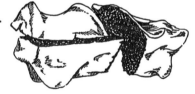

C.

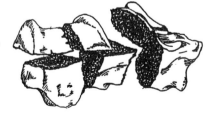

D.

CLASSIFICATION OF OPEN FRACTURES

(Gustilo Classification)

I.   LOW ENERGY WOUND THAT IS USUALLY LESS THAN 1 CM, OFTEN CAUSED BY BONE PIERCING THE SKIN

II. WOUND GREATER THAN 1 CM IN LENGTH WITH MODERATE AMOUNT OF SOFT TISSUE DAMAGE SECONDARY TO HIGHER ENERGY

III. HIGH ENERGY WOUND THAT IS USUALLY GREATER THAN 1 CM WITH EXTENSIVE SOFT TISSUE DAMAGE

Certain factors always constitute a Type III open fracture: high velocity gunshot wound, shotgun wound, segmental fracture, concommitant major vascular injury, significant diaphyseal bone loss, fracture occurring in a farmyard environment or by the crushing of a fast moving vehicle.

Type III fractures are further subdivided into IIIA (limited periosteal muscle stripping with adequate soft tissue coverage), IIIB (extensive soft tissue and periosteal stripping without adequate local coverage), and IIIC (associated with arterial injury requiring repair).

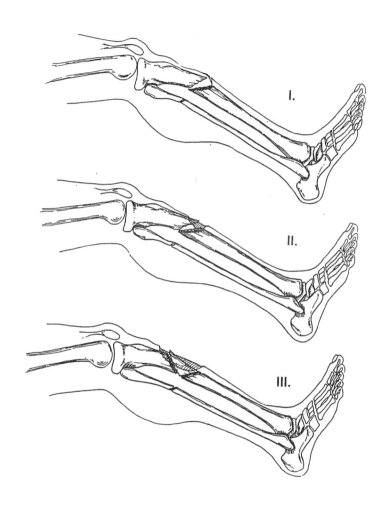

I.

II.

III.

PEDIATRICS

PHYSEAL INJURIES

(Modified Salter-Harris Classification)

I.   COMPLETE SEPARATION OF THE EPIPHYSIS FROM THE METAPHYSIS WITHOUT EVIDENCE OF METAPHYSEAL FRAGMENT

II. FRACTURE PROPAGATES ACROSS THE GROWTH PLATE FOR A DISTANCE AND EXITS THROUGH THE METAPHYSIS

III. FRACTURE PROPAGATES ACROSS THE GROWTH PLATE AND EXITS THROUGH THE EPIPHYSIS CAUSING AN INTRA-ARTICULAR FRACTURE

IV. VERTICAL FRACTURE THAT IS INTRA-ARTICULAR AND TRAVERSES THROUGH THE EPIPHYSIS, ACROSS THE GROWTH PLATE, AND METAPHYSIS

V.   CRUSH INJURY TO THE GROWTH PLATE

VI. PERIPHERAL INJURY TO THE EDGE OF THE PHYSIS OR PERICHONDRAL RING

Type II is the most common fracture configuration. Metaphyseal fragmant is referred to as Thurston Holland fragment.

All growth plate fracrures require anatomic reduction to decrease chances of growth arrest.

Type V is rare.

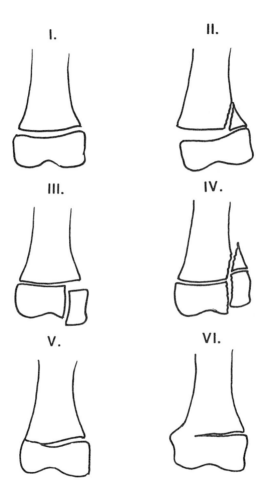

I.

II.

III.

IV.

V.

VI.

SUPRACONDYLAR FRACTURES OF THE HUMERUS

(Pirone Classification)

I. UNDISPLACED

II. PARTIAL DISPLACEMENT WITH CONTACT BETWEEN PROXIMAL
     AND DISTAL FRAGMENTS

    A. POSTERIOR TILT

    B. POSTERIOR TRANSLATION

III. COMPLETE DISPLACEMENT WITHOUT CONTACT BETWEEN THE
      PROXIMAL AND DISTAL FRAGMENTS

The same classification scheme is applicable to flexion type supracondylar fractures.

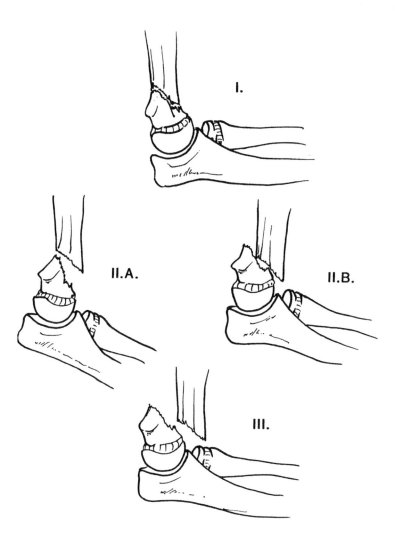

I.

II.A.

II.B.

III.

LATERAL CONDYLE FRACTURE

(Milch Classification)

I.   FRACTURE LINE BEGINS IN THE METAPHYSIS, CROSSES THE PHYSIS, AND THROUGH THE EPIPHYSIS LATERAL TO THE TROCHLEA GROOVE

II.   FRACTURE ORIGINATES IN THE METAPHYSIS, TRAVERSES THE PHYSIS, AND EXITS INTO THE TROCHLEAR REGION

Ossification center of the lateral condyle extends into the trochlea.

Type II is more common and represents a Salter-Harris II fracture pattern.

Type I is uncommon and represents a Salter-Harris IV fracture pattern.

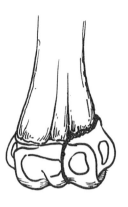

I.

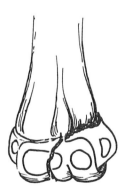

II.

173

MEDIAL CONDYLE FRACTURE

(Milch Classification)

I. FRACTURE LINE ORIGINATES IN THE METAPHYSIS AND TRAVERSES
    THROUGH THE TROCHLEA NOTCH

II. FRACTURE TRAVERSES FROM THE METAPHYSIS INTO THE
    CAPITOTROCHLEAR GROOVE

Type I is more common.

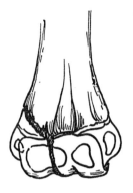

I.

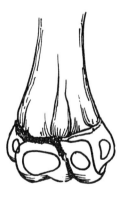

II.

FRACTURES OF THE PROXIMAL RADIUS

(Wilkins Classification)

I.   SALTER-HARRIS I OR II FRACTURE OF THE PROXIMAL RADIUS PHYSIS

II.   SALTER-HARRIS IV FRACTURE OF THE PROXIMAL RADIUS PHYSIS

III. METAPHYSEAL FRACTURE ONLY, WITHOUT PHYSEAL INJURY

I and II are the most common fracture patterns.

May occur with elbow dislocation.

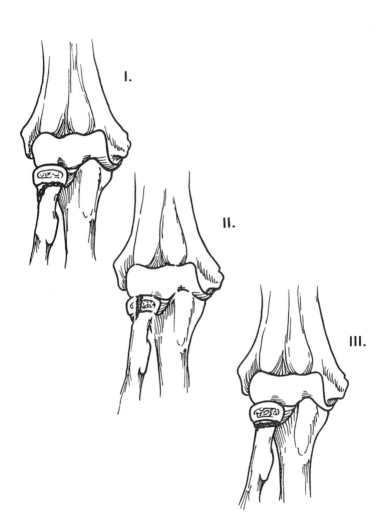

I.

II.

III.

INJURIES TO THE ACRIOMIOCLAVICULAR JOINT

(Dameron and Rockwood Classification)

I.   MILD SPRAIN WITHOUT DISRUPTION OF THE PERIOSTEUM

II. PARTIAL DISRUPTION OF THE DORSAL PERIOSTEUM
     WITH SOME ABNORMAL DISTAL CLAVICLE MOBILITY

III. DISRUPTION OF THE DORSAL PERIOSTEUM WITH GROSS
     INSTABILITY OF THE DISTAL CLAVICLE

IV. DISRUPTION OF THE PERIOSTEUM AND DISTAL CLAVICLE
     POSTERIOR INTO, AND OCCASIONALLY, THROUGH THE
     TRAPEZIUS MUSCLE

V.   SEVERE DISRUPTION OF THE PERIOSTEUM AND DISTAL CLAVICLE
     TO A SUBCUTANEOUS POSITION

VI. DISTAL CLAVICLE DISPLACED BENEATH THE COROCOID PROCESS

Acriomioclavicular and coracoclavicular ligaments remain attached to the periosteum of the clavicle.

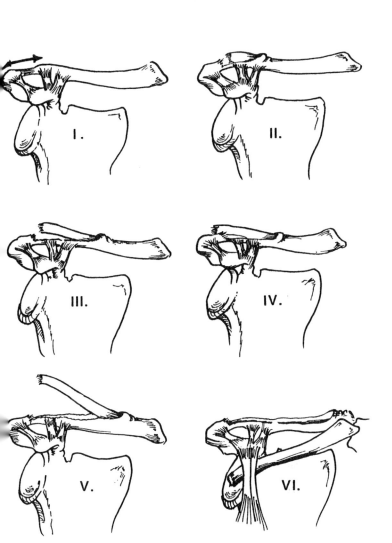

ATLANTOAXIAL ROTATORY DISPLACEMENT

(Fielding Classification)

I.   SIMPLE ROTATORY DISPLACEMENT WITH ANTERIOR SHIFT
     OF THE FIRST CERVICAL VERTEBRAE (C1)

II. ROTATORY DISPLACEMENT OF C1 WITH AN ANTERIOR SHIFT
     OF 5 MM OR LESS

III. ROTATORY DISPLACEMENT OF C1 WITH AN ANTERIOR SHIFT
     OF GREATER THAN 5 MM

IV. ROTATORY DISPLACEMENT OF C1 WITH A POSTERIOR SHIFT

Type I is the most common.

I.

II.

III.

IV.

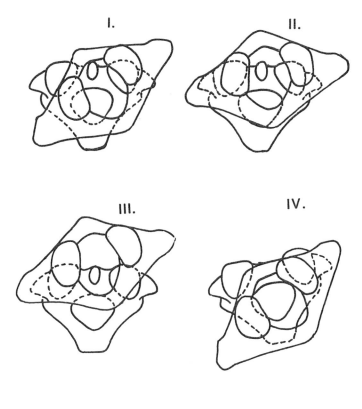

HIP FRACTURES

(Delbet and Colonna Classification)

I.   TRANSEPIPHYSEAL FRACTURES — THROUGH THE GROWTH PLATE

II. TRANSCERVICAL FRACTURES — BETWEEN THE EPIPHYSEAL PLATE
     AND THE BASE OF THE NECK

III. CERVICOTROCHANTERIC FRACTURE — BASE OF THE FEMORAL NECK

IV. INTERTROCHANTERIC OR PERITROCHANTERIC

Type II is the most common.

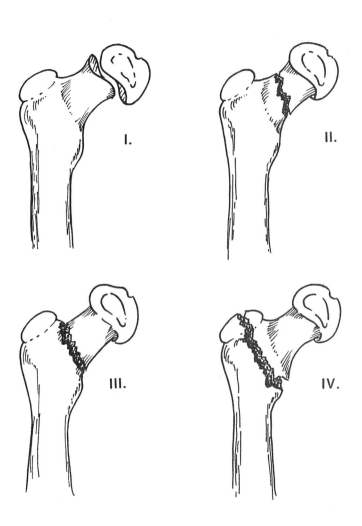

AVULSIONS OF THE TIBIAL TUBERCLE

(Watson Jones Classification)

I. TIBIAL TUBERCLE AVULSED AND HINGED UPWARD WITHOUT
    DISPLACEMENT OF THE BASE

II. TIBIAL TUBERCLE AVULSED AND HINGE FRACTURES WITH
    RETRACTION IN A PROXIMAL DIRECTION

III. TIBIAL TUBERCLE AND PORTION OF THE ARTICULAR SURFACE
     INCLUDED

Type III is a Salter-Harris IV fracture.

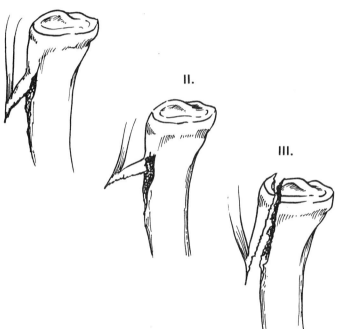

I.

II.

III.

DISTAL TIBIA AND FIBULA PHYSEAL FRACTURES

(Dias and Tachdjian Classification)

I.   SUPINATION — EXTERNAL ROTATION (SER)

II.   PRONATION — EVERSION AND EXTERNAL ROTATION (PEER)

III.   SUPINATION — PLANTAR FLEXION (SPF)

IV.   SUPINATION — INVERSION (SI)

V.   AXIAL COMPRESSION

VI.   JUVENILE TILLAUX

VII.   TRIPLANE

VIII.   OTHER

Combines the Lauge-Hansen principles and the Salter-Harris classification.

The first word in the classification represents the foot position and the second phrase indicates the direction of the disrupting force.

Reduction maneuver is accomplished by reversing the disrupting force.

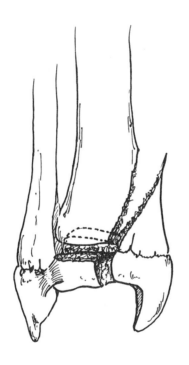

187

DISTAL TIBIA AND FIBULA PHYSEAL FRACTURES

(Dias and Tachdjian Classification)

I.   SUPINATION — EXTERNAL ROTATION (SER)

       STAGE I. SALTER-HARRIS I OR II WITH LONG SPIRAL DISTAL
                    TIBIAL METAPHYSEAL LOCATED POSTERIORLY

       STAGE II. SPIRAL FRACTURE OF THE FIBULA OR SALTER-HARRIS
                    FRACTURE

I.

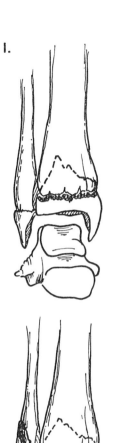

Stage

I.

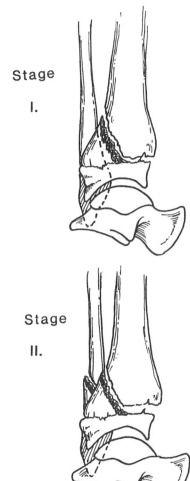

Stage

II.

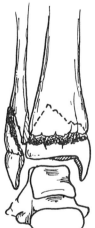

189

DISTAL TIBIA AND FIBULA PHYSEAL FRACTURES

(Dias and Tachdjian Classification)

II. PRONATION — EVERSION AND EXTERNAL ROTATION (PEER)

  SALTER-HARRIS II FRACTURE OF THE TIBIA WITH SHORT
    FIBULAR FRACTURE 4 TO 7 CM FROM THE LATERIAL
    MALLEOLUS

III. SUPINATION — PLANTAR FLEXION (SPF)

  SALTER-HARRIS II FRACTURE OF THE DISTAL TIBIA VISUALIZED
    ON LATERAL X-RAY

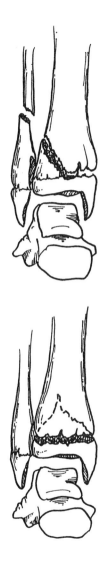

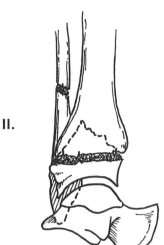

II.

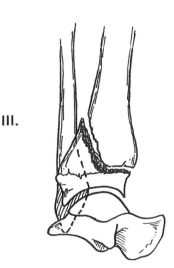

III.

DISTAL TIBIA AND FIBULA PHYSEAL FRACTURES

(Dias and Tachdjian Classification)

IV. SUPINATION — INVERSION (SI)

STAGE I. SALTER-HARRIS I OR II FRACTURE OF THE
DISTAL FIBULA PHYSIS FROM TRACTION

STAGE II. SALTER-HARRIS III OR IV THE DISTAL MEDIAL
TIBIA

IV.

Stage

I.

Stage

II.

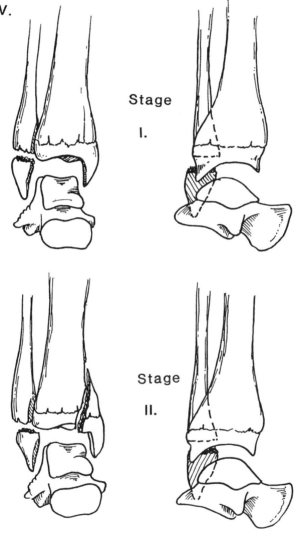

193

DISTAL TIBIA AND FIBULA PHYSEAL FRACTURES

(Dias and Tachdjian Classification)

V.   AXIAL COMPRESSION

DIRECT LOAD TO THE TIBIAL PHYSIS

V.

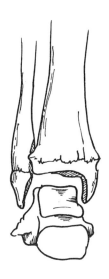
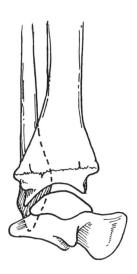

DISTAL TIBIA AND FIBULA PHYSEAL FRACTURES

(Dias and Tachdjian Classification)

VI.   JUVENILE TILLAUX

      ISOLATED FRACTURE OF THE LATERAL PART OF THE
      DISTAL TIBIA PHYSIS, A SALTER-HARRIS III FRACTURE

VI.

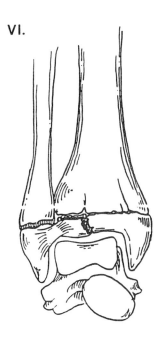

DISTAL TIBIA AND FIBULA PHYSEAL FRACTURES

(Dias and Tachdjian Classification)

VII.   TRIPLANE

FRACTURE PATTERN IN 3 PLANES WITH 3 FRAGMENTS.

ONE FRAGMENT IS THE ANTEROLATERAL PORTION OF THE DISTAL
TIBIA, A SALTER-HARRIS III FRACTURE

THE SECOND FRAGMENT IS THE REMAINDER OF THE PHYSIS AND
THE POSTERIOR SPIKE OF THE DISTAL TIBIA METAPHYSIS,
A SALTER-HARRIS II FRACTURE

THE THIRD FRAGMENT IS THE REMAINDER OF THE DISTAL TIBIAL
METAPHYSIS AND SHAFT

VII.

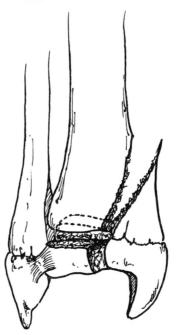

OSTEONECROSIS AND OSTEOCHONDROSIS

I.   **BASE OF PHALANGES**
             (THIEMANN)

II.   **METACARPAL HEAD**
             (MAUCLAIRE)

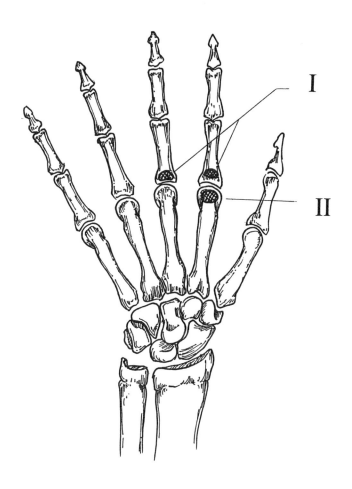

I

II

203

I. SCAPHOID
    (PREISER)

II. LUNATE
    (KIENBÖCK)

III. DISTAL ULNA
    (BURNS)

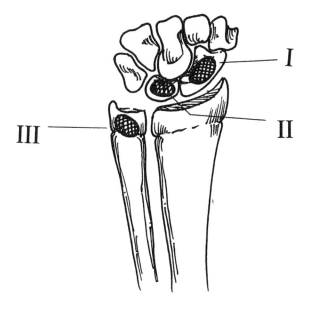

I.   PRIMARY OSSIFICATION CENTER
         (KÖHLER)

II. SECONDARY OSSIFICATION CENTER
         (SINDING-LARSEN)

III. TIBIA TUBERCLE
     (OSGOOD-SCHLATTER)

IV. MEDIAL PROXIMAL
         (BLOUNT)

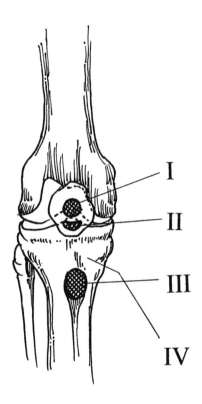

I

II

III

IV

I.   **DISTAL TIBIA**
                (LIFFERT-ARKIN)

II.   **TALUS**
                (DIAZ)

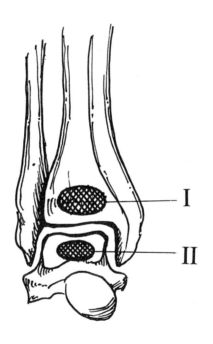

I

II

I.   **VERTEBRAL DISC**
     (SCHMORL-BEADLE)

II. **VERTEBRAL BODY**
         (CALVÉ)

III. **VERTEBRAL EPIPHYSIS**
         (SCHEUERMANN)

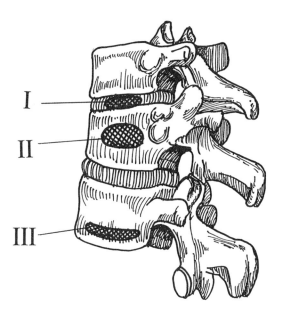

I.   FEMORAL EPIPHYSIS
        (LEGG- CALVÉ-PERTHES)

II.   GREATER TROCHANTER
        (MANDL)

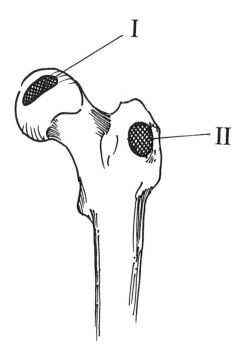

I. ILIAC CREST
(BUCHMAN)

II. ISCHIAL APOPHYSIS
(MILCH)

III. ISCHIOPUBIC SYNCHONDROSIS
(VAN NECK)

IV. SYMPYSIS PUBIS
(PIERSON)

214

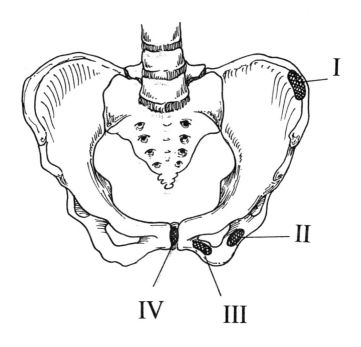

I

II

IV   III

I.   NAVICULAR
     (KÖHLER)

II. SECOND METATARSAL
     (FRIEBERG)

III. FIFTH METATARSAL
     (ISELIN)

IV. CALCANEUS APOPHYSIS
     (SEVER)

216

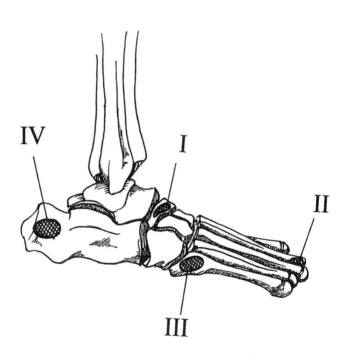

I. HUMERAL HEAD
    (HASS)

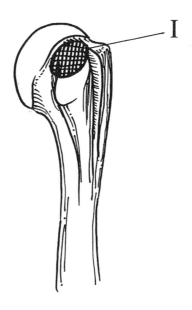

I

I.   CAPITELLUM
      (PANNER)

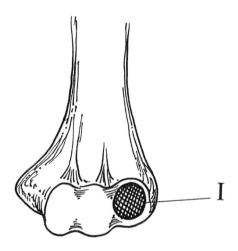

I

221

EPONYMS

AVIATOR'S ASTRAGALUS

Implies a variety of fractures of the talus; described after World War I as rudder bar is driven into foot during a plane crash.

BARTON'S FRACTURE

Displaced articular lip fracture of the distal radius; may be associated with carpal subluxation. Fracture configuration may be in a dorsal or volar direction.

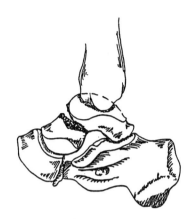

Aviator's Astragalus

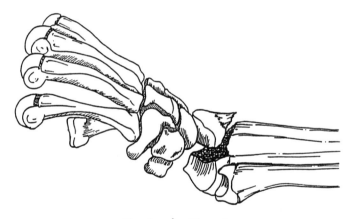

Barton's Fracture

BENNETT'S FRACTURE

Oblique fracture of the first metacarpal base separating a small triangular volar lip fragment from the proximally displaced metacarpal shaft.

BOSWORTH FRACTURE

Fracture of the distal fibula with fixed displacement of the proximal fragment posteriorly behind the posterolateral tibial ridge.

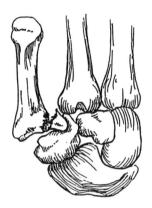

Bennett's Fracture

Bosworth Fracture

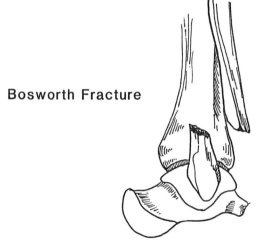

BOXER'S FRACTURE

Fracture of the fifth metacarpal neck with volar displacement of the metacarpal head.

BURST FRACTURE

Fracture of the vertebral body from axial load, usually with outward displacement of the fragments. May occur in cervical, thoracic, or lumbar spine.

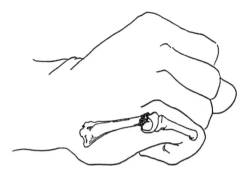

Boxer's Fracture

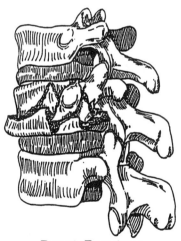

Burst Fracture

CHANCE FRACTURE

Distraction fracture of the thoracolumbar vertebral body with horizontal disruption of the spinous process, neural arch, and vertebral body.

CHAUFFEUR'S FRACTURE (HUTCHINSON'S FRACTURE)

Oblique fracture of the radial styloid, initially attributed to the starting crank of an engine being forcibly reversed by a backfire.

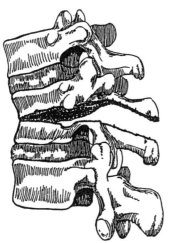

Chance Fracture

Chauffeur's
Fracture

(Hutchinson's
Fracture)

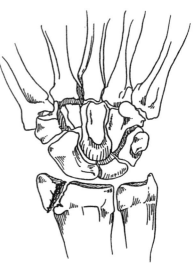

231

CHOPART'S FRACTURE and DISLOCATION

Fracture and/or dislocation involving Chopart's joints (talonavicular and calcaneocuboid joints) of the foot.

CLAY-SHOVELER'S (COAL-SHOVELER'S) FRACTURE

Spinous process fracture of the lower cervical or upper thoracic vertebrae. Injury initially attributed to workers attempting to throw upwards a full shovel of clay, but the clay adhered to the shovel causing a sudden flexion force opposite to the neck musculature.

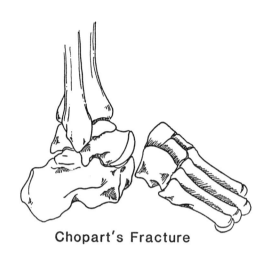

Chopart's Fracture

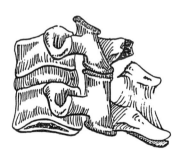

Clay Shoveler's (Coal Shoveler's)
Fracture

COLLES' FRACTURE

General term for fractures of the distal radius with dorsal displacement, with or without an ulnar styloid fracture. See Frykman's classification for further details.

COTTON'S FRACTURE

Trimalleolar ankle fracture with fractures of both malleoli and posterior lip of the tibia.

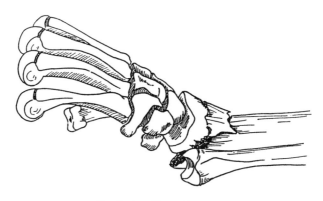

Colle's Fracture

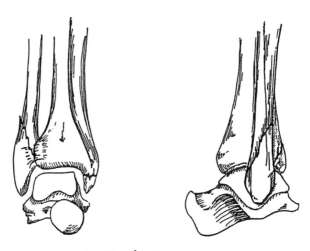

Cotton's Fracture

235

COZEN'S FRACTURE

Proximal tibia metaphyseal fracture that develops valgus deformity.

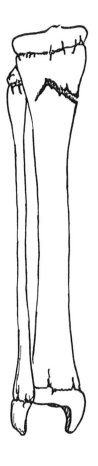

237

DIE PUNCH FRACTURE

Intra-articular distal radius fracture with impaction of the dorsal aspect of the lunate fossa.

DUPUYTREN'S FRACTURE

Fracture of the distal fibula with rupture of the distal tibiofibular ligaments and lateral displacement of the talus.

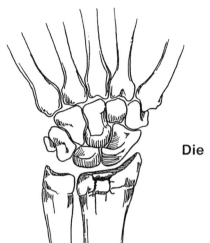

Die Punch Fracture

Dupuytren's Fracture

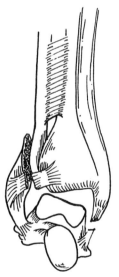

239

DUVERNEY'S FRACTURE

Fracture of the iliac wing without disruption of the pelvic ring.

ESSEX - LOPRESTI'S FRACTURE

Radial head fracture with associated dislocation of the distal radioulnar joint.

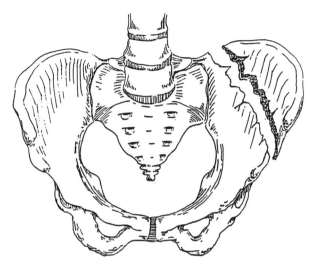

Duverney's Fracture

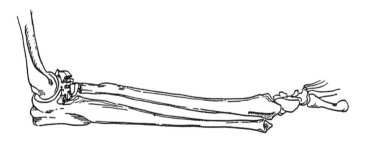

Essex-Lopresti's Fracture

GALEAZZI'S FRACTURE

Fracture of the radius in the distal third associated with subluxation of the distal ulna.

GREENSTICK FRACTURE

Incompletely fractured bone in a child, with a portion of the cortex and periosteum remaining intact on the compression side of the fracture.

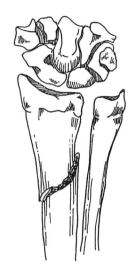

Galeazzi's Fracture

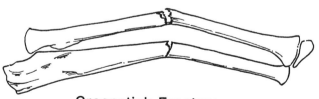

Greenstick Fracture

HAHN - STEINTHAL FRACTURE

Fracture of the capitellum involving a large osseous portion and may involve adjacent trochlea. See classification section for further details of capitellum fractures.

HANGMAN'S FRACTURE

Fracture through the neural arch of the second cervical vertebrae (axis).

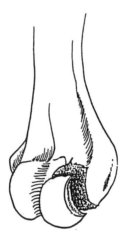

Hahn-Steinthal Fracture

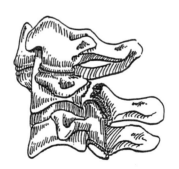

Hangman's Fracture

245

HILL - SACHS FRACTURE

Posterolateral humeral head compression fracture caused by anterior glenohumeral dislocation and impaction of the humeral head against the anterior glenoid rim.

HOLSTEIN - LEWIS FRACTURE

Fracture of the distal third of the humerus with entrapment of the radial nerve.

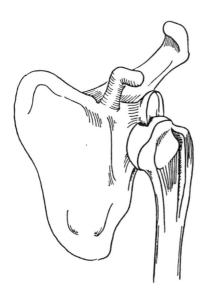

Hill–Sachs Fracture

Holstein–Lewis Fracture

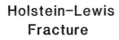

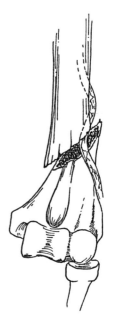

HUTCHISON'S FRACTURE

See CHAUFFEUR'S FRACTURE, pp 208 - 209.

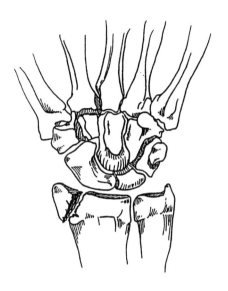

Hutchinson's Fracture

JEFFERSON'S FRACTURE

Comminuted fracture of the ring of the atlas due to axial compressive forces. Fractures usually occur anterior and posterior to the lateral facet joints.

JONES FRACTURE

Diaphyseal fracture of the base of the fifth metatarsal.

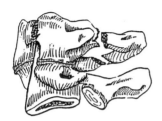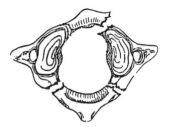

Jefferson's Fracture

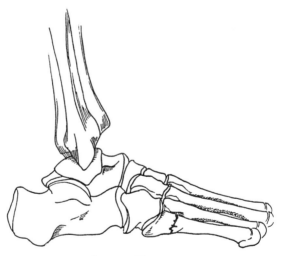

Jones Fracture

KOCHER - LORENZ FRACTURE

Slice fracture of the capitellum involving articular cartilage with minimal subchondral bone. See classification section for further details of capitellum fractures.

LISFRANC'S FRACTURE DISLOCATION

Fracture and/or dislocation involving Lisfranc's (tarsometatarsal) joint of the foot. Lisfranc was one of Napoleon's surgeons and described traumatic foot amputation through the tarsometatarsal joint level.

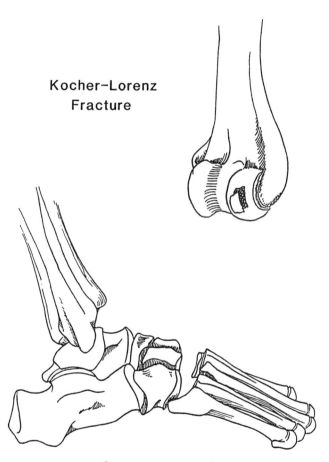

Kocher–Lorenz
Fracture

Lisfranc's Fracture Dislocation

LEFORT-WAGSTAFFE FRACTURE

Avulsion fracture of the anterior fibula tubercle caused by the anterior tibiofibular ligament.

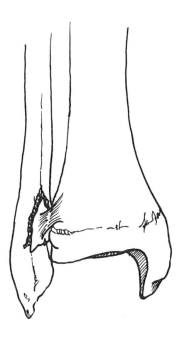

MAISONNEUVE'S FRACTURE

Fracture of the proximal fibula with syndesmosis rupture and associated medial malleolus fracture or deltoid ligament rupture.

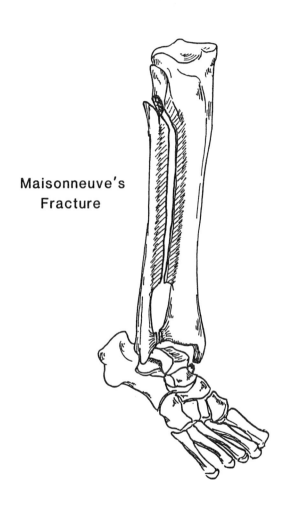

Maisonneuve's
Fracture

MALGAIGNE'S FRACTURE

Unstable pelvic fracture with vertical fractures anterior and posterior to the hip joint.

MALLET FINGER

Flexion deformity of the distal interphalangeal joint caused by extensor tendon separation from the distal phalanx. The deformity may be secondary to direct injury of the extensor tendon or an avulsion fracture from the dorsum of the distal phalanx where the tendon inserts.

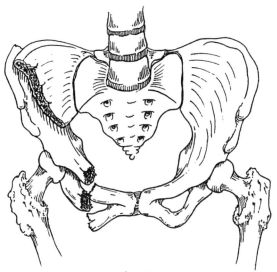

Malgaigne's Fracture

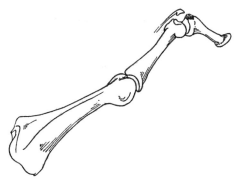

Mallet Finger

MONTEGGIA'S FRACTURE

Fracture of the proximal third of the ulna with associated dislocation of the radial head. Fracture complex has been further classified by Bado; see classification section.

NIGHTSTICK FRACTURE

Isolated fracture of the ulna secondary to direct trauma.

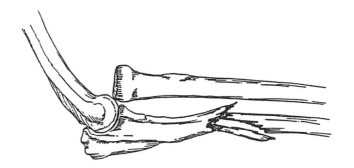

Monteggia's Fracture

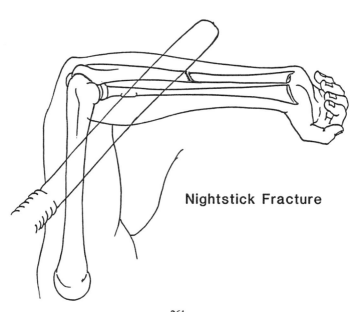

Nightstick Fracture

261

POSADAS' FRACTURE

Transcondylar humerus fracture with displacement of the distal fragment anteriorly and dislocation of the radius and ulna from the bicondylar fragment.

POTT'S FRACTURE

Fracture of the fibula within 2 to 3 inches above the lateral malleolus with rupture of the deltoid ligament and lateral subluxation of the talus. Pott did not describe disruption of the tibiofibular ligaments.

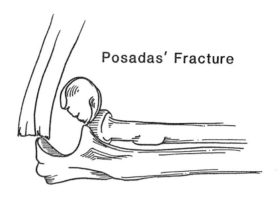

Posadas' Fracture

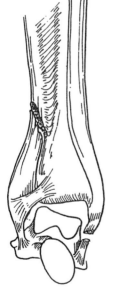

Pott's Fracture

263

ROLANDO'S FRACTURE

Y-shaped intra-articular fracture of the thumb metacarpal.

SEGOND'S FRACTURE

Avulsion fracture of the lateral tibial condyle from the bony insertion of the iliotibial band.

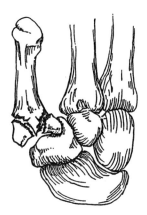

Rolando's Fracture

Segond's Fracture

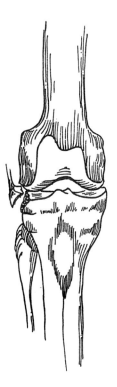

265

SHEPHERD'S FRACTURE

Fracture of the lateral tubercle of the posterior talar process.

SMITH'S FRACTURE

Fracture of the distal radius with palmar displacement of the distal fragment. Also referred to as a reverse Colles' fracture.

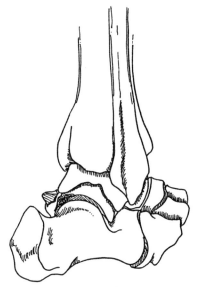

Shepherd's Fracture

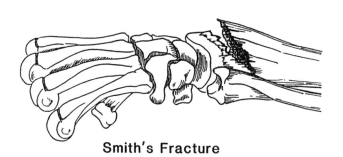

Smith's Fracture

STIEDA'S FRACTURE

Avulsion fracture of the medial femoral condyle at the origin of the medial collateral ligament.

STRADDLE FRACTURE

Bilateral fractures of the superior and inferior pubic rami.

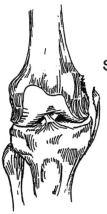

Stieda's Fracture

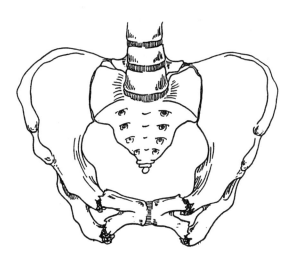

Straddle Fracture

269

THURSTON HOLLAND FRAGMENT

Metaphyseal fragment that occurs with a Salter-Harris II growth plate injury.

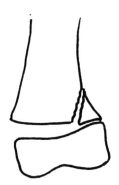

TEARDROP FRACTURE

Flexion fracture dislocation of the cervical spine with associated triangular anterior fragment of the involved vertebrae. Injury complex is unstable with posterior ligamentous disruption.

TILLAUX'S FRACTURE

Fracture of the lateral half of the distal tibial physis during differential closure of the physis. The medial part of the tibial physis has already fused.

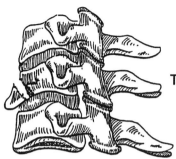

Teardrop Fracture

Tillaux's Fracture

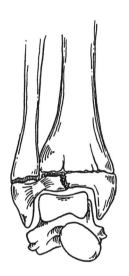

273

TILLAUX-CHAPUT FRACTURE

Avulsion fracture of the anterior lateral tibial margin caused by the anterior tibiofibular ligament.

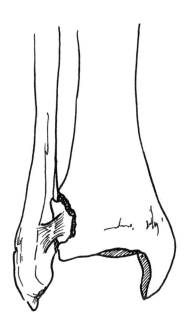

TODDLER'S FRACTURE

Spiral fracture of the tibia in infants and children, usually caused by low energy torsional forces.

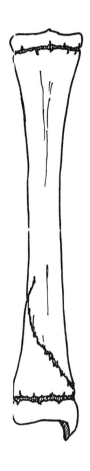

277

TRIPLANE FRACTURE

Fracture in 3 planes with 3 fragments.

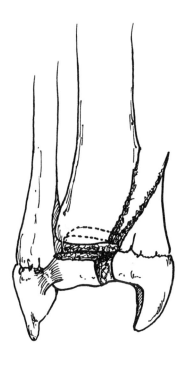

TORUS FRACTURE

Impaction fracture of childhood as the bone buckles instead of fracturing completely.

WALTHER'S FRACTURE

Ischioacetabular fracture which passes through the pubic rami and extends toward the sacroiliac joint. The medial wall of the acetabulum is displaced inward.

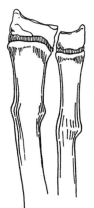

Torus Fracture

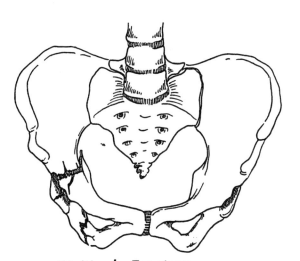

Walther's Fracture

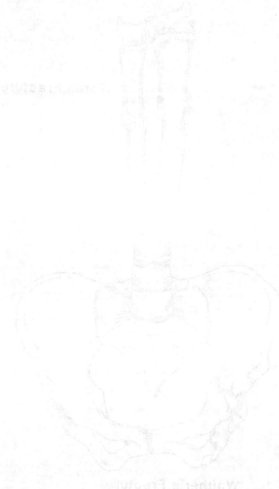

282

REFERENCES

Anderson, H.G.: *The Medical and Surgical Aspects of Aviation*, Oxford University Press, London, 1919.

Anderson, L.D.: "Fractures of the Shafts of the Radius and Ulnar, In Rockwood, C.A., and D.P. Green (Eds.), *Fractures in Adults, Second Edition*, J.B. Lippincott, Philadelphia, 1983, pp. 511-558.

Anderson, L.D., and R.T. D'Alonzo: "Fractures of the Odontoid Process of the Axis," *J. Bone Joint Surg.* 46A: 310-233, 1970.

Ashurst, A.P.C.: "An Anatomical and Surgical Study of Fractures of the Lower End of the Humerus," *The Samuel D. Gross Prize Essay of the Philadelphia Academy of Surgery, 1910*, Lea and Febiger, Philadelphia, 1910.

Bado, J.L.: "The Onteggia Lesion," *Clin. Orthoped.* 50: 71-86, 1967.

Barton, J.R.: "Views and Treatment of an Important Injury to the Wrist," *Med. Examiner* 1: 365, 1838.

Baumann, J.U., and R.D. Campbell, Jr.: "Significance of Architectural Types of Fractures of the Carpal Scaphoid and Relation to Timing of Treatment," *J. Trauma* 2: 431-438, 1962.

Bennett, E.H.: "Fractures of the Metacarpal Bones," *Dublin J. Med. Sci.* 73: 72-75, 1882.

Bosworth, D.M.: "Fracture Dislocation of the Ankle with Fixed Displacement of the Fibula Behind the Tibia," *J. Bone Joint Surg.* 29: 130-135, 1947.

Brower, A.C.: *Orthopaedic Ranks North America* vol 14, No.19: pp332, 1983

Bryan, R.S.: "Fractures About the Elbow in Adults," *AAOS Instructional Course Lectures* 30: 200-223, 1981.

Bryan, R.S., and B.F. Morrey: "Fractures of the Distal Humerus," In Morrey, B.F. (Ed.), *The Elbow and Its Disorders*, W.B. Saunders, Philadelphia, 1985, pp. 325-327.

Bucholz, R.W., K. and Gill: "Classification of Injuries of the Thoracolumbar Spine," *Orthoped. Clin. North. Am.* 17: 67-73, 1986.

Cancelmo, Jr., J.J.: "Clay-Shoveler's Fracture. A Helpful Diagnostic Sign," *Am. J. Roentgenol.* 115: 540, 1972.

Cass, J.R.: "Fractures and Dislocations Involving the Midfoot," In Chapman, M.W. (Ed.), *Operative Orthopaedics.* J.B. Lippincott, Philadelphia, 1988, pp. 1737-1755.

Chance, C.Q.: "Note on a Type of Flexion Fracture of the Spine," *Br. J. Radiol.* 21: 452-453, 1948.

Chaput, V.: *Fractures Mallolaires du Cou-de-pied et les Accidents du Travail*, Paris, Masson and Cie, 1907.

Chapman, M.W. (Ed.): *Operative Orthopaedics*, J.B. Lippincott, Philadelphia, 1988.

Chutro, P.: *Fractures de la Extremidad Inferior Del Humero en los Ninos.* Theses J. Peuser, Buenos Airs, 1904.

Colles, A.: "On the Fracture of the Carpal Extremity of the Radius," *Edinburg. Med. Surg. J.* 10: 182-186, 1814.

Colonna, P.C.: "Fractures of the Neck of the Femur in Childhood. A Report of Six Cases," *Ann. Surg.* **88**: 902, 1928.

Colton, C.L.: "Fractures of the Olecranon in Adults: Classification and Management," *Injury* **5**: 121-129, 1973-74.

Cotton, F.J.: "A New Type of Ankle Fracture," *J. Am. Med. Assoc.* **64**: 318-321, 1915.

Cozen, L.: "Fracture of the Proximal Portion of the Tibia in Children Followed by a Valgus Deformity," *Surg. Gynec. Obstet.* **97**: 183-188, 1953.

Dameron, T.B., and C.A. Rockwood: "Fractures and Dislocations of the Shoulder," In Rockwood, C.A., K.E. Wilkins, and R.E. K.E., King (Eds.), *Fractures in Children*, J.B. Lippincott, Philadelphia, **1984**, pp. 624-653.

DeLee, J.S.: "Fractures and Dislocations of the Foot," In Mann, R.A. (Ed.), *Surgery of the Foot*, C.V. Mosby, St. Louis, 1986, pp. 592-714.

Denis, F.: "The Three Column Spine and Its Significance in the Classification of Acute Thoracolumbar Spinal Injuries," *Spine* **8**: 817-831, 1983.

Denis, F., S. Davis, and T. Comfort: "Sacral Fractures: An Important Problem," *Clin. Orthoped.* **227**: 67-81, 1988.

DePalma, A.F.: *The Management of Fractures and Dislocations*, W.B. Saunders, Philadelphia, 1959.

Destot, E.: *Injuries of the Wrist*, Ernest Benn, London, 1925.

Dias, L.S.: "Fractures of the Tibia and Fibula," In Rockwood, C.A., and D.P. Green, (Eds.), *Fractures in Children*, J.B. Lippincott, Philadelphia, 1984, pp. 983-1042.

Dias, L.S., and M.O. Tachdjian: "Physeal Injuries of the Ankle in Children," *Clin. Orthoped*, **136**: 230-233, 1978.

Dimon, J.H., and J.S. Hughston: "Unstable Intertrochanteric Fractures of the Hip," *J. Bone Joint Surg.* **49A**: 440-450, 1967.

Dunbar, J.S., H.F. Owen, M.B. Nogrady, and R. MeLesse: "Obscure Tibial Fracture of Infants - The Toddler's Fracture," *J. Can. Assoc. Radiol.* **25**: 136-144, 1964.

Dupuytren, G.: "Of Fractures of the Lower Extremity of the Fibula, and Luxations of the Foot," Reprinted In: *Medical Classics* **4**: 151-172, 1939.

Duverney, J.G.: *Traite des Maladies des Os*. Volume 1, DeBure L'Aine', 1751.

Edwards, H.C.: "Mechanism and Treatment of Backfire Fracture," *J. Bone Joint Surg.* **8**: 701-717, 1926.

Essex-Lopresti, P.: "Fractures of the Radial Head with Distal Radio-ulnar Dislocation. Report of Two Cases," *J. Bone Joint Surg.* **33B**: 224-247, 1951.

Essex-Lopresti, P.: "Results of Reduction in Fractures of the Calcaneum," *J. Bone Joint Surg.* **33B**: 284, 1951.

Essex-Lopresti, P.: "The Mechanism, Reduction Techniques, and Results in Fractures of the Os Calcis," *Br. J. Surg.* **39**: 395-419, 1952.

Fielding, J.W., and R.J. Hawkins: "Atlanto-axial Rotatory Fixation," *J. Bone Joint Surg.* **59A**: 37-44, 1977.

Frykman, G.: "Fractures of the Distal Radium Including Sequelae - Shoulder, Hand, Finger Syndrome, Disturbance in the Distal Radio-Ulnar Joint and Impairment of Nerve Functions," *Acta Orthoped. Scand.* **Suppl. 108**: 1-153, 1967.

Galeazzi, R.: "Uber ein Besonderes Syndrom bei Verlrtzunger im Bereich der Unter Armknochen," *Arch. Orthop. Unfallchir.* **35**: 557-562, 1934.

Garden, R.S.: "Stability and Union in Subcapital Fractures of the Femur," *J. Bone Joint Surg.* **46B**: 630-647, 1964.

Green, D.P., and E.T. O'Brien: "Fractures of the Thumb Metacarpal," *Southern Med. J.* **65**: 807-814, 1972.

Green, D.P., and S.A. Rowland: "Fractures and Dislocations in the Hand," In Rockwood, C.A., D.P. Green (Eds.), *Fractures in Adults, Second Edition*, J.B. Lippincott, Philadelphia, 1984, pp. 313-410.

Gustilo, R.B., R.M. Mendoza, and D.N. Williams: "Problems in the Management of Type III (Severe) Open Fractures. A New Classification of Type III Open Fractures," *J. Trauma* **24**: 742-746, 1984.

Hahn, N.F.: "Fall von eine Besonderes Varietat der Frakturen des Ellenbogens," *Zeitschrift Qundarzte und Geburtshelte* **6**: 185-189, 1853.

Harris, J.H., B. Edeiken-Monreo, and D.R. Kopaniky: "A Practical Classification of Acute Cervical Spine Injuries," *Orthoped. Clin. North Am.* **17**: 15-30, 1986.

Hawkins, L.G.: "Fractures of the Neck of the Talus," *J. Bone Joint Surg.* **47A**: 1170-1175, 1965.

Heckman, J.D.: "Fractures and Dislocations of the Foot," In Rockwood, C.A., and D.P. Green (Eds.), *Fractures in Adults, Second Edition*, J.B. Lippincott, Philadelphia, 1984, pp. 1703-1832.

Hill, H.A., and M.D. Sachs: "The Grooved Defect of the Humeral Head. A Frequently Unrecognized Complication of Dislocations of the Shoulder Joint," *Radiology* **35**: 690-700, 1940.

Holland, C.T.: "A Radiographic Note on Injuries to the Distal Epiphysis of the Radius and Ulna," *Proc. Royal Soc. Med.* **22**: 695-700, 1929.

Holstein, A., G.B. Lewis: "Fractures of the Humerus with Radial Nerve Paralysis," *J. Bone Joint Surg.* **45A**: 1382, 1963.

Holdsworth, F.W.: "Fractures, Dislocations, and Fracture-dislocations of the Spine," *J. Bone Joint Surg.* **45B**: 6-20, 1963.

Hoppenfield, S., P. deBoer: *Surgical Exposures in Orthopaedics. The Anatomic Approach*, J.B. Lippincott, Philadelphia, 1984, p. 507.

Ideberg, R.: "Fractures of the Scapula Involving the Glenoid Fossa," In Bateman, J.E., and R.P. Welsh (Eds.), *Surgery of the Shoulder*, B.C. Becker, New York, 1984, pp. 63-66.

Jefferson, G.: "Fracture of Atlas Vertebrae: Report of Four Cases, and a Review of Those Previously Recorded," *Br. J. Surg.* **7**: 407-422, 1920.

Johnston, G.W.: "A Follow-up of One Hundred Cases of Fracture of the Head of the Radius with a Review of the Literature," *Ulster Med. J.* **31**: 51-56, 1962.

Jones, R.: "Fracture of the Base of the Fifth Metatarsal Bone by Indirect Violence," *Ann. Surg.* **35**: 697-700, 1902.

Kaplan, L.: "The Treatment of Fractures and Dislocations of the Hand and Fingers. Technic of Unpadded Casts for Carpal, Metacarpal and Phalangeal Fractures," *Surg. Clin. North Am.* **20**: 1695-1720, 1940.

Kocher, T.: *Beitrage zur Kenntniss Einiger Tisch Wichtiger Frakturforman*, Sallman, Basel, 1896, pp. 585-591.

Kyle, R.F., R.B. Gustilo, and R.F. Premer: "Analysis of 622 Intertrochanteric Hip Fractures: A Retrospective and Prospective Study," *J. Bone Joint Surg.* **61A**: 216-221, 1979.

Lauge-Hansen, N.: "Ligamentous Ankle Fractures: Diagnosis and Treatment," *Acta. Chir. Scan.* **97**: 544-550, 1949.

LeFort, L.: "Note sur une Variete non Decrete de Fracture Verticale de la Malleole Esterne par Arrachement," *Bull. Gen. Ther.* **110**: 193-199, 1886.

Lorenz, H.: "Zur Kenntniss der Fraktura Humeri (Eminentiae Capitate)," *Deutsche Zeitschr. f. Chir.* **78**: 531-545, 1905.

Maisonneuve, J.B.: "Recherches sur la Fracture du Perone," *Arch. Gen. Med.* **7**: 165-187, 433-473, 1840.

Malgaigne, J.F.: *Treatise on Fractures*, J.B. Lippincott, Philadelphia, 1959.

Mason, J.A., and N.M. Shutkin: "Immediate Active Motion Treatment of Fractures of the Head and Neck of the Radius," *Surg. Gynecol. Obstet.* **76**: 731-737, 1943.

Meyers, M.H., and F.M. McKeever: "Fractures of the Intercondylar Eminence of the Tibia," *J. Bone Joint Surg.* **52A**: 1677-1684, 1970.

Milch, H.: "Fractures and Fracture Dislocations of the Humeral Condyles," *J. Trauma* **4**: 592-607, 1964.

Monteggia, G.B.: *Instituzioni Chirrugiche, Volume 5*, Maspero, Milan, 1814.

Morrey, B.F.: *The Elbow and Its Disorder*, W.B. Saunders, Philadelphia, 1985.

Muller, M.E., M. Allgower, R. Schneider, and H. Willenegger: *Manual of Internal Fixation, Second Edition*, Springer-Verlag, New York, 1979.

Neer, C.S., II: "Displaced Proximal Humeral Fractures: I. Classification and Evaluations," *J. Bone Joint Surg.* **52A**: 1077-1089, 1970.

Neer, C.S., II: "Fractures of the Distal Third of the Clavicle," *Clin. Orthoped.* **58**: 43-50, 1968.

Ogden, J.A.: "The Uniqueness of Growing Bones," In Rockwood, C.A., K.E. Wilkens, and R.E. King (Eds.), *Fractures in Children*, J.B. Lippincott, Philadelphia, 1984, pp. 1-86.

Pantazopoulus, T., P. Galanos, P., E. Voganas, *et al.*: "Fractures of the Neck of the Talus," *Acta. Orthoped. Scand.* **45**: 296-306, 1974.

Pipkin, G.: "Treatment of Grade IV Fracture-Dislocation of the Hip," *J. Bone Joint Surg.* **39A**: 1027-1042, 1957.

Pirone, A.M., H.K. Graham, and J.I. Krajbich: "Management of Displaced Extension-type Supracondylar Fractures of the Humerus in Children," *J. Bone Joint Surg.* **70A**: 641-650, 1988.

Pott, P.: *Some Few General Remarks on Fractures and Dislocations*, Hawes, Clarks, Collins, London, 1768.

Quenu, E. and G. Kuss: "Etude sur les Luxations du Metatarse (Luxations Metatarso-Transiennes) due Diastasis entre le I. et le Metatarsien," *Rev. Chir. (Paris)*, **39**: 281-336, 720-791, 1093-1134, 1909.

Rang, M.: *The Growth Plate and Its Disorders*, Williamsand Wilkins, Baltimore, 1969.

Regan, W., and B. Morrey: "Fractures of the Coronoid Process of the Ulna," *J. Bone Joint Surg.* **71A**: 1348-1354, 1989.

Resnick, D., and Niwayama, G.: *Diagnosis of Bone and Joint Disorders, Second Edition*, W.B. Saunders, Phiadelphia, 1988 Chapters 82 & 84

Riseborough, E.J., and E.L. Radin: "Intercondylar T Fractures of the Humerus in the Adult," *J. Bone Joint Surg.* **51A**: 130-141, 1969.

Roberts, J.B., and J.A. Kelly: *Treatise on Fractures, Second Edition*, J.B. Lippincott, Philadelphia, 1921.

Rockwood Jr., C.A., and D.P. Green (Eds.): *Fractures in Adults, Second Edition*, J.B. Lippincott, Philadelphia, 1984.

Rolando, S.: "Fracture de la Base du Premier Metcarpien: Et Principalement sur une Variete non Encore Decrits," *Presse Med.* 33: 303, 1910.

Ruedi, T., and M. Allgower: "Fractures of the Lower End of the Tibia into the Ankle Joint," *Injury* 1: 92, 1969.

Russe, O.: "Fracture of the Carpal Navicular: Diagnosis, Non-operative Treatment, and Operative Treatment," *J. Bone Joint Surg.* 42A: 759-768, 1960.

Salter, R.B., and W.R. Harris: "Injuries Involving the Epiphyseal Plate," *J. Bone Joint Surg.* 45A: 587-622, 1963.

Schatzker, J.: "Compression in the Surgical Treatment of Fractures of the Tibia," *Clin. Orthoped.* 105: 220-239, 1974.

Scheck, M." "Long Term Follow Up of Treatment of Comminuted Fractures of the Distal End of the Radius by Transfixion with Kirschner Wires and Case," *J. Bone Joint Surg.* 44A: 337-351, 1962.

Schneider, R.C., and E.A. Kahn: "Chronic Neurological Sequelae of Acute Trauma to the Spine and Spinal Cord. Part I. The Significance of the Acute Flexion or "Teardrop" Fracture-dislocation of the Cervical Spine," *J. Bone Joint Surg.* 38A: 985-997, 1956.

Segond, P.: "Rechershes Cliniques et Experimentaelis sur les Epanchements Sanquins du Genou par Entorse," *Prog. Met. (Paris)* 7: 297, 1879.

Seinsheimer, F.: "Subtrochanteric Fractures of the Femur. *J. Bone Joint Surg.* 60A: 300-306, 1978.

Shepherd, F.J.: "A Hitherto Undescribed Fracture of the Astragalus," *J. Anat. Physiol.* 18: 79-81, 1882.

Smith R.W.: *A Treatise on Fractures in the Vicinity of Joints, and on Certain Forms of Accidental and Congenital Dislocation*, Hodges and Smith, Dublin, 1854.

Stark, H.H., J.H. Bayes, and J.N. Wilson: "Mallet Finger," *J. Bone Joint Surg.* 44A: 1061-1068, 1962.

Steinthal, D.: "Die Isolierte Fraktur der Eminentia Capitat in Ellenbogengelenk," *Centrallbl. f. Chirugi* 15: 17-20, 1898.

Stieda, A.: *Arch. f. Klin. Chir.* 85: 815, 1908.

Tillaux, P.: *Traite de Chirurgie Clinique*, Vol. 2, Paris, Asselin & Houzeau, 1848.

Tile, M.: "Pelvic Ring Fractures: Should They be Fixed," *J. Bone Joint Surg.* 70B: 1-12, 1988.

Tile, M.: *Fractures of the Pelvis and Acetabulum*, Williams and Wilkins, Baltimore, 1984.

Wagstaffe, W.W.: "An Unusual Form of Fracture of the Fibular," *Saint Thomas Hospital Reports* 6: 43, 1875.

Walther, C.: "Recherches Experimentelles sur Certains Fracturas de la Cavietecotyloide," *Bull. Soc. Anat. Paris* 5: 561, 1891.

Watson-Jones, R.: *Fractures and Joint Injuries, Volume 2, 3rd Edition*, Williams and Wilkins, Baltimore, 1946.

Wilkins, K.E.: "Fractures and Dislocations of the Elbow Region," In Rockwood, C.A., K.E. Wilkins, and R.E. King (Eds.), *Fractures in Children, Third Edition*, J.B. Lippincott, Philadelphia, pp. 509-828, 1991.

Winquist, R.A., S.T. Hansen, Jr., and D.K. Clawson: "Closed Intramedullary Nailing of Femoral Fractures: A Report of Five Hundred and Twenty Cases," *J. Bone Joint Surg.* **66A**: 529-539, 1984.

Wood-Jones, F.: "The Examination of Bodies of 100 Men Executed in Nubia in Roman Times," *Br. Med. J.* **1**: 736-737, 1908.

Wood-Jones, F.: "The Ideal Lesion Produced by Judicial Hanging," *Lancet* **1**: 53, 1913.

INDEX

ORDER FORM FOR HANDBOOKS

TITLE	Price x Quantity
Handbook of Commonly Prescribed Drugs, 15thEdition (2000) ISBN # 0-942447-35-2	$18.95 x ____ = $ ____.___
Handbook of Common Orthopaedic Fractures, 4th Edition (2000) ISBN # 0-942447-36-0	$18.95 x ____ = $ ____.___
Travelers Guide to International Drugs - Western Hemisphere Year 2000 ISBN # 0-942447-30-1	$8.95 x ____ = $ ____.___
Travelers Guide to International Drugs - European Edition, Volume 1 (2000) ISBN # 0-942447-33-6	$8.95 x ____ = $ ____.___
Travelers Guide to International Drugs - European Edition, Volume 2 (2000) ISBN # 0-942447-34-4	$8.95 x ____ = $ ____.___
Travelers Guide to International Drugs, **European Vol. I & II (2000) **Package** *A savings of $2.00*	$15.90 x ____ = $ ____.___
Drug Charts in Basic Pharmacology, 2nd Edition (1998) ISBN # 0-942447-26-3	$18.00 x ____ = $ ____.___
Warning: Drugs in Sports, 1st Edition (1995) ISBN # 0-942447-16-6	$14.50 x ____ = $ ____.___
Handbook of Commonly Prescribed Pediatric Drugs, 6th Edition (1999) ISBN # 0-942447-27-1	$18.50 x ____ = $ ____.___
Antimicrobial Therapy in Primary Care Medicine, 1st Edition ISBN # 0-942447-22-0	$17.00 x ____ = $ ____.___
Shipping and Handling Charges (see below) **PA Residents: Add 6% Sales Tax**	Sub-Total = $ ____.___ = $ ____.___ = $ ____.___ Total = $ ____.___

Shipping and Handling Charges:

Add $6.00 for orders between $10.00 and $49.99

Add $8.50 for orders between $50.00 and $99.99

Add $10.50 for orders between $100.00 and $149.99

Add $12.50 for orders greater than $150.00

For mail orders for Handbooks, please complete the reverse side of this form.

ORDER FORM FOR TEXTBOOK
IN PHARMACOLOGY

TITLE	PRICE x QUANTITY		
Basic Pharmacology in Medicine, Fourth Edition (1995), 880 pages ISBN 0-942447-04-2	$ 49.95 x ____ = $ ____.____		
	SUB-TOTAL	=	$ ____.____
Shipping and Handling		=	$ 5.50
PA Residents: Add 6% Sales Tax		=	$ ____.____
	TOTAL	=	$ ____.____

Send mail orders for Handbooks or Textbook to:

MEDICAL SURVEILLANCE INC.
P.O. Box 480   Willow Grove, PA 19090

(PLEASE PRINT)

Name_____Degree_____

Organization_____

Street Address_____

City_____State_____Zip_____

Telephone Number_____

Payment: Check____ VISA____ MC____ Discov____ Am. Express____

Credit Card No._____ Exp. Date_____

Signature_____

FOR FURTHER INFORMATION CALL: 800 - 417-3189 or 215 - 784-0976
FAX: 215 - 657-1475

REQUEST FOR INFORMATION

If you wish to be placed on a mailing list for information concerning new publications and updates, please fill out the form below and mail to:

MEDICAL SURVEILLANCE INC.
P.O. Box 480   Willow Grove, PA 19090

(PLEASE PRINT)

Name_____

Organization_____

Street Address_____

City_____State_____

Zip Code_____

Telephone Number (Optional)_____

FOR FURTHER INFORMATION CALL:
800 - 417-3189 or 215 - 784-0976

E-Mail us at **medsurveillance@aol.com**

Visit Us on the **World Wide Web** at
hhtp://www.medicalsurveillance.com